Controlled Explosions in Mental Health

Have you ever wondered why your brain self-sabotages? Or why your actions seem self-defeating or destructive? This book explores how our brains have evolved to favour survival over mental well-being – creating 'controlled explosions' – and provides practical ways to understand, acknowledge and defuse them.

Controlled Explosions in Mental Health identifies everyday scenarios in which one may experience self-destructive behaviour such as procrastination or self-criticism. Each chapter guides the reader through key examples of controlled explosions, identifying and exploring their possible functions. Readers will learn how to identify when one or more of these 'explosions' are operating in their lives, recognise the potential harm or difficulties this may cause, and learn practical ways to navigate and overcome. The friendly, accessible narrative, teamed with illustrations, guided examples, and worksheets to aid self-practice, makes this book the ultimate companion for navigating your mental health.

This book supports the path to self-awareness, helping the reader take control of their own struggles with insight, care, and compassion. It's a must-read for any reader looking to better understand their mental health and well-being.

Dr Charlie Heriot-Maitland is a clinical psychologist, researcher, author, and trainer. Having started his career as a therapist in NHS mental health services, he co-founded an organisation in 2012 called Balanced Minds, which specialises in providing Compassion Focused Therapy (CFT) and self-help resources for the public, and CFT training and consultation for professionals and organisations.

'As a leading expert in Compassion Focused Therapy approaches, Charlie Heriot-Maitland offers an impactful model for understanding, and addressing, common behaviors such as self-sabotage, self-criticism, and self-harm. This accessible book provides insights and tools that individuals can apply to their own experiences through a compassionate lens.'

Kate Hardy, *Clinical Professor, Department of Psychiatry and Behavioral Sciences, Stanford University, USA.*

'One of the most common questions we ask ourselves is: why do I feel like this? There are of course a range of answers to do with things that happened to us in the past, things that are happening around us now, and how we are dealing with them. Less commonly do we recognise that we have brains that have all kinds of built-in biases, problems and glitches. Our potentials to feel anxious, angry, depressed, love and hate exist within us because we have evolved brain systems that enable or allow them. Most of us are unaware of just how much our evolved brain circuits are ticking away in the background. After all, how many of us wake up in the morning and decide to have a panic attack? Or just for the hell of it have a depression, a rage attack, or start becoming paranoid with our friends? Nobody! These just get triggered and take us over.

This wonderful book by one of the leading international authorities on evolution and compassion focused approaches to psychotherapy guides us into a deep understanding about how our brains are set up for some of the distressing experiences we have. The more we understand the nature of our brains, become mindful of processes operating within us, and how we can engage in ways of thinking or acting that can make these distressing states worse or more manageable, the more we can work with them rather than against them. Dr Heriot-Maitland provides a highly accessible tour of the challenges of the mind and what we can do to help. Full of wisdoms, stories, empathic reflections and guides for compassionate working with a very tricky brain.'

Paul Gilbert OBE, *Professor at University of Derby, President and Founder of the Compassionate Mind Foundation, UK.*

'Empowering, wise, and deeply human, *Controlled Explosions in Mental Health* is a lifeline for anyone trying to break free from cycles of pain and self-blame. A beautiful invitation to meet yourself with kindness and a must-read for anyone ready to heal from within and build a more supportive, resilient relationship with themselves, this is one of those special books that doesn't just offer insight – it also offers hope.'

Eleanor Longden, *Postdoctoral Service User Research Manager at Greater Manchester Mental Health NHS Foundation Trust, UK.*

'Compassion Focused Therapy is one of the best ways for us to reframe and re-contextualise our mental world and Charlie is one of its greatest practitioners and researchers. In this book he lays out a new way of understanding the parts of ourselves that turn inwards and sometimes work against us and, by putting this within an evolutionary context, he helps us work through these tendencies in a judgement-free way. I have no doubt that those who read this book will come away with more self-awareness and more self-compassion and pretty much nothing is more important than that.'

Russell Razzaque, *Consultant Psychiatrist, Director of R&D NELFT, Bye Fellow Cambridge University, Clinical & Strategic Director National Collaborating Centre for Mental Health, Lead for Compassionate & Relational Care RCPsych, UK.*

'This book skilfully blends Charlie's extensive clinical wisdom and knowledge of the science of compassion to create a practical, accessible guide to deepening self-awareness. This book is a must for anyone wishing to explore and bring compassion to the understandable but potentially self-defeating life patterns.'

Kate Lucre, *Consultant Psychotherapist, Birmingham and Solihull Mental Health Foundation Trust, UK.*

'Dr Charlie Heriot-Maitland has done it again, bringing warmth, clarity and deep clinical wisdom to one of the trickiest topics in mental health. *Controlled Explosions* offers a powerful metaphor for the ways we self-sabotage, criticise, and even harm ourselves—not because we're broken, but because we're trying, however imperfectly, to protect ourselves. With compassion at its core, this book invites us to better understand these internal processes and begin responding to them with courage, kindness and care. A must-read for anyone who's ever wondered, "Why do I do this to myself?" and wants to find a gentler, wiser way forward.'

Stan Steindl, *Clinical Psychologist at Psychology Consultants Pty Ltd and Adjunct Professor at The University of Queensland, Australia.*

'Charlie has robustly and creatively extended a metaphor for self-criticism into a framework that really helps us connect with the nuances of how this shows up for us. His usual attention to detail and readable style makes this book great for both clinicians and the general public. Instead of self-sabotaging, let's move towards a compassionate analysis of its evolved protective function and onwards to addressing our fears in ways that can lead to more rewarding lives.'

Angela Kennedy, *Founder & Director of*
Trauma Informed Community Action CIC and
Independent Consultant at Innovating for Wellbeing, UK.

Controlled Explosions in Mental Health

A Compassionate Guide to Understanding Why Our Brains Self-Sabotage, Self-Criticise, and Self-Harm

Charlie Heriot-Maitland

Routledge
Taylor & Francis Group
LONDON AND NEW YORK

Designed cover image: Alfie Heriot-Maitland

First published 2026
by Routledge
4 Park Square, Milton Park, Abingdon, Oxon OX14 4RN

and by Routledge
605 Third Avenue, New York, NY 10158

Routledge is an imprint of the Taylor & Francis Group, an informa business

© 2026 Charlie Heriot-Maitland

For Product Safety Concerns and Information please contact our EU representative GPSR@taylorandfrancis.com. Taylor & Francis Verlag GmbH, Kaufingerstraße 24, 80331 München, Germany.

British Library Cataloguing-in-Publication Data
A catalogue record for this book is available from the British Library

ISBN: 978-1-032-90818-2 (hbk)
ISBN: 978-1-032-90815-1 (pbk)
ISBN: 978-1-003-55992-4 (ebk)

DOI: 10.4324/9781003559924

Typeset in Times New Roman
by KnowledgeWorks Global Ltd.

Contents

Acknowledgements

I owe a great deal to the many people who have sat down with me, over the past 20 years of being a mental health worker and therapist, to courageously talk with me about their personal lives, fears, traumas, and emotional struggles. I have so appreciated the time spent listening, sharing, and learning with every one of you. To my wife, who has been my love and co-wanderer for 23 years, and our three boys who are reminding us about the marvel of teenage life, and who have always been ready to jump wholeheartedly into our family adventures. My loyal running companion, Dora. My friends and colleagues at Balanced Minds, in the Compassionate Mind community, and in the academic worlds of Stanford, King's, and Glasgow. My collaborators and mentors, in particular a couple of Kates (one in the US, one in the UK) who have been absolute powerhouses of support for me and my work in recent years.

Introduction

In March 2015, a 5-foot Second World War bomb was found in Bermondsey, London, and was driven a few miles out of the city to a quarry in North Kent for a timed, controlled explosion at 9am.

An important job of any Police bomb disposal unit – or 'bomb squad', as they're commonly known – is to intentionally explode or disrupt a bomb under controlled conditions to avert the greater risk that could occur if the device was to explode at some other (unknown) time.

Some of the controlled explosions used by bomb squad officers are designed to intentionally detonate the explosive material of a bomb in a controlled environment, so the blast occurs, and the gases are safely released from the chemical materials inside. Other controlled explosions intentionally disrupt the structure and components of a device so that its main explosive material is not detonated. Both are examples of intentional and targeted destruction of something to prevent a (bigger) harm from occurring.

Of course, controlled explosions are also used for other purposes beyond Police or military bomb squads. They are also used to destroy suspicious substances and to demolish unsafe buildings, towers, bridges, and other structures. Again, these are very targeted and strategic 'attacks' on something that ultimately reduce the risk of even greater harm and damage.

Controlled explosions in mental health

In this book, we will delve into the complex and intriguing area of human experience where some of the things we do to ourselves and our lives (often automatically, and unconsciously) may have quite serious unintended consequences for our mental health and well-being.

This book uses the concept of *controlled explosions* as a metaphor to explore a key psychological process that we each encounter from time to time, and to varying degrees, in our daily lives. Our brains often generate self-directed harms and problems as a protective strategy against other anticipated threats from happening. Essentially, we create harms and problems to ourselves in order to avoid or prevent some other (greater) anticipated harm.

DOI: 10.4324/9781003559924-1

There is a range of examples of how this shows up in our lives, from day-to-day examples that we can all relate to, to more extreme versions that can emerge after particularly difficult and traumatic experiences, to those which may relate to mental health conditions. The chapters of this book will shine a light across the broad range. This is not with the aim of providing a comprehensive account of every single example, but more to convey that these experiences occur on a continuum throughout the whole population. As readers of this book, there will be relevance for each of your lives, whether it's around your day-to-day procrastinating and sabotaging of daily tasks, your self-criticism, or whether you have experienced more distressing versions of self-harm and injury. Observing these on a continuum might help us to understand each other a bit more, and to understand some of the common themes in our human struggles.

Which versions do you notice in your life?

These are some of the typical questions and concerns that people have, which really make them start to wonder why they are their own worst enemy. Are any of these familiar to you?

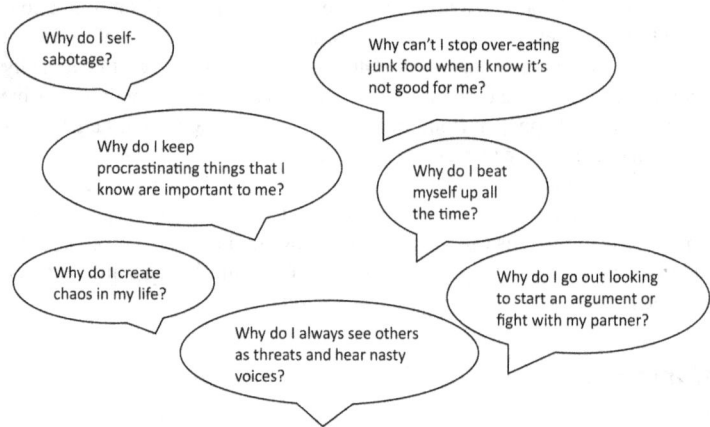

Why do I self-sabotage?

Why can't I stop over-eating junk food when I know it's not good for me?

Why do I keep procrastinating things that I know are important to me?

Why do I beat myself up all the time?

Why do I create chaos in my life?

Why do I go out looking to start an argument or fight with my partner?

Why do I always see others as threats and hear nasty voices?

Common questions and concerns

Have you ever asked yourself questions like this? Are there other versions of this in your life? The chapters of this book will be packed full of examples, so as we go through these together, you may start to notice some patterns of self-sabotage that you hadn't even realised were there before. You may start to understand a bit more about what's been holding you back in your life, or what's been keeping you stuck, for example, with work, your health, or with your relationships. The more you become aware of your own *controlled explosions*, and the more you start to understand why they are there, the more choices and opportunities you will have in the future for transforming and growing your life in the direction you want.

So why do we have brains that self-sabotage?

Well, that's the big question isn't it! And that question's probably exactly what brought you here to this book. And that's why I'm here too. We're all here because of our shared interest in this perplexing issue of why we humans feel things, perceive things, and do things that are self-defeating. We all appear to have versions of this to some degree or other, and what's so curious about this is that, on the surface, these patterns only seem to bring harm and problems our way. Are we all the unfortunate victims of mis-firing neurons? Evolutionary glitches? Or are our neurons firing exactly as they should, but for a reason not yet obvious to us? I am delighted that you have chosen to come on this exploratory journey with me, and I hope these chapters we are about to walk through together will spark the same kind of interest, curiosity, and enlightenment for you as they have done for me.

At the heart of our exploration will be the central idea that our brains may have developed ways of generating self-inflicted problems as a method of avoiding other anticipated threats from happening. Essentially, we create harms and problems to ourselves to prevent some other (greater) anticipated harm or problem.

Consider this choice:

*   Option 1 – the possibility of an out-of-control (unknown) threat
*   Option 2 – the certainty of a controlled (known) threat

It's a difficult choice because neither option is very good. But what is the least bad option? As we will learn in Chapter 1, our brains have a tendency towards caution and overestimating danger and will often favour the certainty (option 2) over uncertainty (option 1). There is something comforting for us about the familiar and known. Anything to avoid the unknown.

In daily life, this might take the form of self-sabotaging behaviour, where we find various ways of derailing our own progress and creating barriers to achieving our goals. Another example is self-criticism, which can range from self-critical focus on our inadequacies, to more distressing forms such as self-attacking and self-hating. Some of us might self-punish and physically self-harm or find other ways of bringing suffering upon ourselves. These forms of self-inflicted suffering are a major burden on our well-being. Some versions of self-harm many of us will be doing, even if we wouldn't use that term for it; for example, we may be restricting food, punishing our body with exercise or sex, biting our fingernails, or picking our skin. Referring to these as 'controlled explosions' implies that while they are indeed damaging to us on one level, there may be some greater harms that they are functioning to protect us from. In this book, we will be exploring the possible function of such experiences.

To delve deeper into the question of *why* we self-inflict these things, it might be helpful to further unpack exactly what it is we are asking: *"why might it be functional to have a brain that can self-generate its own threat?"* Or we could equally approach this from the other angle, on the threat-receiving side. In the controlled explosion scenario, our brain is (simultaneously) both the giver *and* receiver of an explosion. So, while one part of us is creating the harm or threat, another part is responding in a protective way or activating a protective response. So, the equivalent and equally valid question would be: *"why might it be functional to have a brain that can self-stimulate its own protective responses?"*

This second question might be easier to answer, because, from an evolutionary perspective, it could be very helpful and adaptive to have ways of switching on our protective responses. This is perhaps a bit like rehearsing or training, as it could help us prepare for (real) threats in the world. Perhaps this could be a way of getting used to the presence of threat, possibly building more tolerance and mastery over the experience of threat. Our protective responses (such as fight, flight, freeze, submit, dissociate) are also getting a bit of exercise, making them more honed and ready to switch on as and when a 'real' (external) danger comes along.

While training and exercising our threat 'muscles' would be a handy trait at the species level; i.e., for a species to evolve for survival. At the individual level, it may be less so. For example, if our brain regularly creates self-directed threats, we may end up feeling less motivated, more depressed, and more likely to stay at home. So, while switching on these patterns may make sense at the species level of evolution and surviving, it may not at the individual level of well-being, mental health, and thriving. And if we notice that our protective patterns are being overused, at the expense of our life goals and well-being, then we might choose to do something about it.

About this book

This book will guide us through many different examples of controlled explosions and their possible functions. To help understand the various functions and roles, we will personalise these as characters – as if they were parts of us or 'selves' – doing a particular job for us. In keeping with the *controlled explosions* metaphor, these characters will be profiled as members of *the bomb squad*, each performing different types of controlled explosion.

The bomb squad has three units, with five members in each. These units will provide the backbone and structure to the book and will keep us anchored to our central theme of controlled explosions as we cover a wide range of illustrations and examples. The units are:

- The Self-Sabotage Unit, who create explosions that can derail our lives and plans
- The Self-Criticism Unit, who create explosions that can harm us psychologically
- The Self-Harm Unit, who create explosions that can harm us physically.

The use of character metaphors in this book creates an intentionally playful tone. This, however, is in no way to downplay the serious harm and suffering that many of us experience through our controlled explosions. The impact on our mental health is certainly not a light-hearted matter. However, in the 20 years that I have been working directly with people with mental health difficulties, as well as in mental health research and training activities, I have found that playfulness, warmth, and affiliation is often an essential foundation to establish before we can develop the courage to start looking clearly into the nature of our suffering. The light-hearted and playful use of metaphors like 'controlled explosions' and 'the bomb squad' is intended to provide a non-threatening framework to ease us into an understanding of some very complex and distressing experiences. If this book were to dive straight into heavy, distressing language from the off, there's a good chance that the threat-protective systems in our brains would either resist or disengage us from the topic before we'd even started.

If you are interested in finding out more about the background story of how I came into developing and using the *controlled explosions* metaphor, I have shared an account of this in Appendix 1, along with some other background information about the key influences on my ideas and approach (particularly from the psychology pioneers, Paul Gilbert and Carl Jung).

Ultimately, this book is about supporting self-awareness, self-understanding, and self-help. By encompassing a continuum of examples, from day-to-day to more extreme, this book will be relevant for a broad range of readers, from those who are interested in their daily mental health and well-being, to those who are struggling with mental health difficulties and perhaps receiving support from therapy and other mental health services. The overall aims of the book are to help you to:

i notice when one or more of these controlled explosions might be operating in your life
ii recognise that although, on the one hand, this may be understandable (or functional) for you, on the other hand, it may also be causing you harm or difficulties
iii improve your understanding so that you can make your own wise choices about how to respond, for example, whether to accept or to address these harms.

Part I

The nature of our evolved brains

Chapter 1

Our brains have evolved to favour survival over mental well-being

Chapter summary

This chapter introduces the idea that there are many processes in our minds that are not particularly helpful or conducive to our mental well-being. This is understandable when we consider the evolutionary context in which our brains and minds have developed. Sometimes, for example, our minds can work in ways that might favour a distorted version of reality, over an accurate 'true' version. Sometimes our minds might bias us towards actions that promote our safety and protection, rather than our happiness and psychological well-being. This chapter will lay the foundation for exploring why we have a brain that's great in many ways, but which can also cause us a great deal of problems. This foundation is key to understanding the central topic of this book – our *controlled explosions*, which are (self-generated) harms in service of avoiding or preventing some (bigger) harm.

Imagine this evolutionary scene: a group of our caveman ancestors are sitting around relaxing by their cave after a long day's hunting. There is a rustle in the bushes. The more cautious members of the group estimate that there's a high chance of threat; maybe it's a snake or lion about to attack. They quickly run to safety and hide. Meanwhile some others in the group – who are slightly more relaxed – think 'ah it's probably just the wind' and settle back down for their afternoon snooze.

Fast-forward 100,000 years and which genes do you think we inherited? The 'better to be safe than sorry' genes, or the 'ah it's probably nothing' ones? The slightly more anxious and paranoid ancestors, who were more likely to *over*-estimate danger are probably the ones who survived and passed on their genes to us. Whereas the slightly more relaxed and chilled-out ancestors are probably the ones who got eaten and did not pass on their genes.

DOI: 10.4324/9781003559924-3

Our brain's relationship with threat

There is a very good evolutionary reason why our brains perceive the world in a biased way. The number of situations where we perceive threat *just in case* will considerably outweigh the situations where there is actually a real threat present. It comes down to simple cost–benefit analysis (see doodle). When there is a real threat, there is obviously a very high benefit to perceiving threat and a very high cost to not perceiving threat. This is a matter of life or death. However, when there is no real threat, there is a fairly low cost of perceiving threat (perhaps the wasted energy of running away unnecessarily), and a fairly low benefit of not perceiving threat (the energy saved).

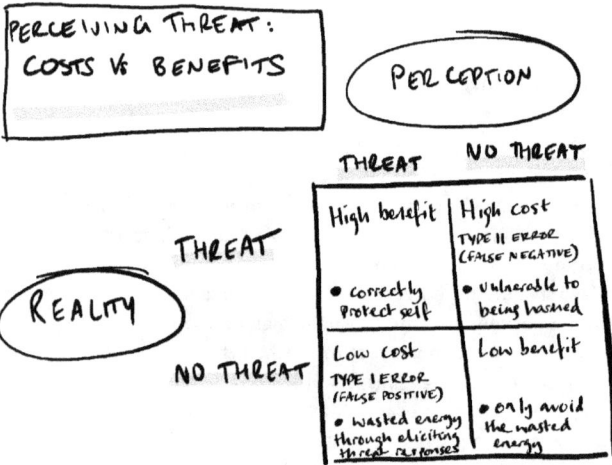

PERCEIVING THREAT: COSTS vs BENEFITS

PERCEPTION

	THREAT	NO THREAT
THREAT (REALITY)	High benefit • correctly protect self	High cost TYPE II ERROR (FALSE NEGATIVE) • vulnerable to being harmed
NO THREAT	Low cost TYPE I ERROR (FALSE POSITIVE) • wasted energy through eliciting threat responses	Low benefit • only avoid the wasted energy

PERCEIVING THREAT HAS EITHER

↑ BENEFIT or ↓ COST

Also, there might be some benefit to the Type I error (false positive) in that you are training (excercising/priming/rehearsing) the protective responses for a future 'real' eventuality.

DOODLE: "Perceiving threat: Costs vs Benefits"[1]

So essentially what this boils down to is that, as humans, we have evolved a brain that favours perceiving threat (even when there isn't one) in order to elicit a protective response in us. We have all inherited a highly sensitive threat-detection and threat-response system. Indeed, if we could attach a suitable tagline or motto for how our evolved brain works, it would be: '*better safe than sorry*'. So that principle makes sense from an evolutionary perspective, where survival is everything, but what does that mean for us, here and now, in our day-to-day lives?

The first thing to consider is how this threat system manifests in human, as opposed to non-human, brains. For humans, another way that our brain has been shaping over hundreds of thousands of years, is in the development of cognitive abilities, such as the ability to use reasoning (for example, attaching meaning to things, such as cause and effect), imagination, planning, and language. We have also developed metacognition, which is the ability to observe, monitor, and control our own cognitive processes (self-monitoring) as well as those of other people (social monitoring). These cognitive capacities are very handy for us as humans, allowing our species to advance, co-operate, and thrive in many wonderful ways. However, there is a trade-off; because the built-in threat bias we all have can actually become even more pronounced, more exaggerated, and more sustained by these (newer) cognitive abilities.

When our threat system is switched on, these aspects of human cognition (imagination, reasoning, metacognition, and so on) can become patterned, co-opted, and utilised by the threat system. For example, if we are experiencing fear in our body, our imagination can become instantly flooded with fear-related predictive scenarios; for example, imagining the worst that could happen. Our reasoning can also become very biased. For example, we create a framework to attach meaning to the fear we're feeling – and often quick and simple reasoning is favoured over more slow nuanced consideration of multiple options. Our planning can become heavily influenced by the *better safe than sorry* principle. With our social- and self-monitoring systems, these are also likely to become enlisted as additional agents for threat protection. For instance, we might start scanning our social world for other people's traits, roles, and movements that could possibly signal threat (perhaps people's dominance, authority, and power), whilst at the same time focusing closely on aspects of ourselves that may signal vulnerability, or may attract harm from others (such as our own weaknesses, flaws, insecurities, or the things we don't like about ourselves). Within our own self-to-self monitoring, it may be that we switch on the parts of ourselves that are threatening (angry, attacking, hostile, and dominant), together with the parts of ourselves that are vulnerable to attack (our exposed flaws and weaknesses).

Stepping back for a minute, let's just think about what's going on here in terms of trade-off, again with reference to our evolutionary cost–benefit analysis. So, on the one hand, from an evolutionary 'survival of the species' perspective, there are many benefits to channelling all our abilities (emotional, attentional, cognitive, behavioural) towards the goal of threat protection. This is how we've evolved. As we've already seen, the benefits of correctly perceiving threat (survival) far outweigh the costs of incorrectly perceiving threat when there is none (wasted energy). So, we throw everything into the possibility that there might be threat, just in case. But have we considered the impact on our mental health? What might be the mental health consequences of flooding our mind with imagined danger scenarios, other people's hostile intentions, and focusing specifically on our flaws and insecurities?

Well of course this causes us a lot of stress and emotional distress. Our advanced cognitive and metacognitive abilities, which help us in so many ways as humans, are now potentially becoming our worst enemies – as far as mental health is concerned. Our human brains have become so advanced that we can create the most terrifying and gruesome scenarios or ideas in our imagination. Think about the scariest horror movie you've seen, or the worst nightmare you've had. We can also use our astute reasoning powers to make a very convincing case to ourselves for why we *should* be terrified. For example, *'my computer did something funny, so it must be that I'm being hacked'*. We then embark on a process of collecting evidence to confirm that belief *('let me scroll the internet for everything that's been written about hackers and scammers')*, which of course strengthens our case for the narrative we've told ourselves. We also use our sophisticated self-to-self monitoring capability to self-criticise and self-attack. We can self-create distress and unpleasant feelings in our own body in service of 'better safe than sorry'. We can create *controlled explosions*.

Let's just pause and take stock of what we've established so far, because this an important starting point and premise for our explorations together in these following chapters – we are recognising that humans have evolved brains that can generate self-directed threats and harms. And in doing so, our brains can essentially stimulate themselves into protective responses. So, one part of us is generating a threat towards us, and another part is receiving this threat. Just think about that – our brain can self-shock, self-attack, and this is all part of evolutionary design. This is not a glitch. This is our brain working exactly as it should – in the interests of survival.

Although our brain's self-generation of problems and harm may well be helpful from the perspective of evolution and survival of our species, it comes at a cost to us at the individual level. And this cost is particularly impactful in the areas of our mental health and well-being. Brains that are geared towards protection are not supposed to give us nice, warm, fuzzy feelings. They're not designed to optimise our happiness. They need to alert us, warn us, shock us. They need to generate in us unpleasant feelings such as fear and disgust. Things that will make us ready and prepared for the many dangers in the world.

The unpleasantness of defences is just part of their utility.
(Randolph Nesse, evolutionary psychiatrist [1])

Before we delve deeper into controlled explosions specifically, I would just like to spend a bit of time introducing you to some of the other quirks of our tricky evolved brain. Do we *really* know what our brains are up to? Do we really appreciate the priorities and principles that govern how our brains function? What if these priorities were not very aligned to our own personal priorities and goals? If so, this is something we should really know about.

Most of us would like to assume that our brain has evolved to work pretty well for what we need it to do. At the very least, we'd like to assume that our brains will provide us with accurate information about the world so that we can make rational decisions about what to do, and how to live our lives. But how accurate is the information that our brain is feeding us? How rational are our decisions? Let's spend a bit of time having a closer look at this brain of ours – this 'helper' we carry around inside our heads – and see what it's *really* up to.

Our brain's relationship with reality

Visual/optical illusions

I have always been intrigued by visual illusions. For me, these are an instant and constant reminder that we can never quite fully believe what we see. Some of my favourite examples appear on page 14. When you look at these illusions you immediately perceive something that you later realise was not real. In example a), the Shepards Table [2], you see two tables that are clearly different shapes and sizes, and its only when you measure them with a ruler, that you discover they are the same size. In example b), the Checkershadow Illusion [3], you see that square A obviously looks a lot darker than square B, but in reality, they are the same shade of grey. In example c), the Skye Blue Café Wall Illusion [4], there is absolutely no doubt that the horizontal lines you are looking at are not parallel. But they are. And even if, after a while, you do manage to convince yourself 100% that they are indeed parallel, you still cannot help but to see non-parallel lines. Thank you, brain – you've been a great help!

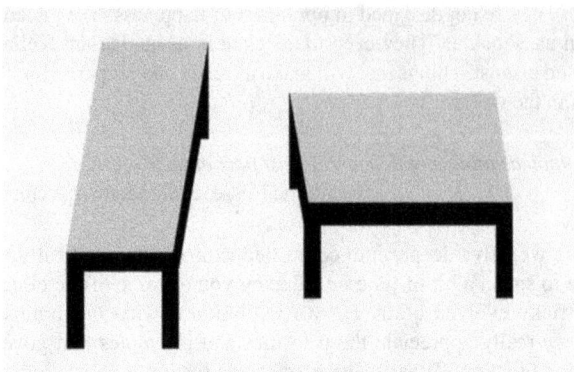

a) The Shepards Table. *Are these two tables the same shape and size?*

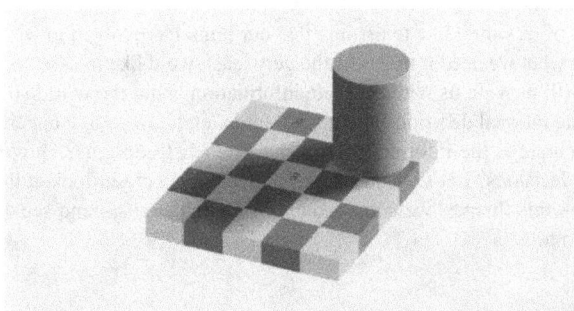

b) The Checkershadow Illusion. *Are squares A & B the same shade of grey?*

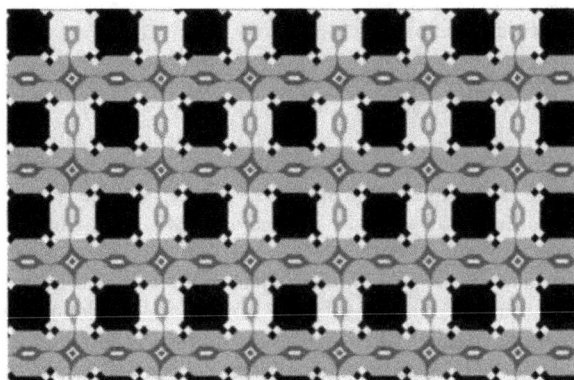

c) The Skye Blue Café Wall Illusion. *Are the horizontal lines all parallel?*

Visual illusion examples

There are many other illusions like this, and if you are interested in searching some of these up, here are the names of a few others:

- the *Lilac Chaser*, otherwise known as the 'Pac-Man' illusion, which demonstrates how our perceptual systems can erase moving dots that we are looking straight at
- the *Train Illusion*, which demonstrates that we can intentionally change our perception of a train's motion, by just using the power of our mind
- the *Dynamic Ebbinghaus*, which demonstrates that we don't directly perceive the size of an object, instead our brain makes inferences (*best guesses*) based on things like the relative sizes of nearby objects
- the *Rice Wave Illusion*, which brilliantly demonstrates that our brain can create the perception of movement in entirely stationary objects
- the *Troxler Effect*, which demonstrates that when our visual system gets bored of what it's looking at, it simply deletes the image from our awareness.

What these visual illusions are showing us is that our brain is making this stuff up! What we see is not necessarily what's there. And yet, even though we can look at hundreds of visual illusions (as I have) and be reminded of this fact time-and-time again, we are still surprised. We are still amazed that our brain could have tricked us in this way. Again! So not only is our brain feeding us its own constructed (hallucinated) version of reality, but it is also intent on covering up this fact and convincing us that it's real. Our brain wants us to remain in a state of being tricked and hoodwinked. It wants us to believe that what we see is the objective reality. It insists that we keep seeing *its* version of the world, not the *real* version, despite all the evidence we might try to gather. However long we spend with our careful ruler measurements of tables and parallel lines, we still see the brain-created version of reality.

Just 10% of the information our brains use to see comes from our eyes.
(Beau Lotto, neuroscientist [5])

Awareness of this can feel quite humbling. To recognise that even with our most advanced powers of rational thinking and logical discernment, there are other powers built deep into this brain of ours that are far greater. Our brain has other guiding principles, such as its evolutionary imperative to survive, that will always override our individual needs for accuracy as well as our personal intentions and goals. Coming to recognise these things could be sobering. It could also be quite disorientating, maybe even scary and uncomfortable. And if that's how you are feeling right now, that's okay and understandable. It's the same for many of us. But as we go through this book together, we will realise that some of these uncomfortable truths can actually be highly liberating for us. Understanding the different pulls and biases in our brains will open up a whole new range of choices for us. As we begin to better understand our brain's reality-distorting tendencies, we will also begin to understand its self-sabotaging tendencies too. We will see that self-sabotage is also linked to unconscious processes and patterns in our brain, some of which relate to personal fears, motives, and needs, and others which relate to evolutionary motives and basic life tasks. Identifying and understanding these (hidden) drivers of our self-directed sabotage, problems, and harms is precisely our mission.

Do we perceive reality?

In an interesting presentation at the TED2015 event, Donald Hoffman invites us to consider the question: *Do we see reality as it is?* [6]. Hoffman uses an evolutionary lens to explain why it is actually very important for our survival fitness to *not* see the world accurately; but instead to see what we need to see in order to survive and reproduce. In that sense, Hoffman argues, our brain gives us a view that is more like an interface (or headset) that actually hides reality and just gives us the snippets of information that will guide our adaptive behaviour. We are talking here about perception itself – the information coming into our awareness – i.e., even before our brain has a chance to unleash all of its other biases, such as with attention and reasoning – the ones we may be more familiar with.

According to Hoffman, it would actually work against us and our ability to survive if we saw all the information accurately. For one, it would overwhelm us. Imagine how much excruciating detail there would be if we had to process every single sensory molecule that was entering into our field of awareness. Not a chance. We need to *construct* a reality that we can deal with, otherwise we'd have no chance of knowing how to navigate the world.

> *"Not seeing the world accurately gives us a survival advantage"*;
> *"What we're seeing is what we need to see to stay alive long enough to reproduce."*
>
> (Donald Hoffman, cognitive psychologist [6])

As we have already seen, the brain has many ways of tricking us. And by evolutionary standards, this is exactly the way it should be. This is a sign that our brain is working perfectly. It is designed (by evolution) to get us to do things that will help us survive and pass on our genes. So our perceptions and actions are often guided by constructions of what is going on in our world, or predictions of what is about to happen, rather than what is actually happening. Some of these ideas are illustrated in another doodle.

DO WE PERCEIVE REALITY?

Evolution does not favour ACCURATE perceptions.

It favours perceptions that will give us the best chance of surviving and reproducing which often requires hiding the truth (objective reality).

OPTICAL ILLUSIONS

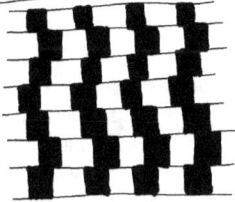

EYES NARROWING

keep myself safe & in control by only allowing snippets of info

SOME EXAMPLES OF SHORTCUTS:

• threat bias (better to be safe than sorry)

• Construct a reality that predicts what might happen next, rather than what is happening now

• Construct a reality based on the minimum information possible to remain shielded from information that could potentially harm

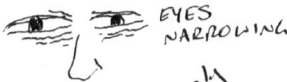

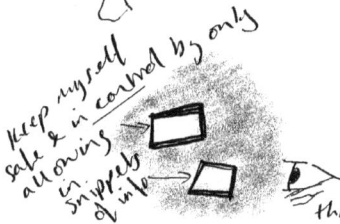

DOODLE: "Do we perceive reality?"

Predictive processing models of perception

Most modern cognitive neuroscientific theories assume there is likely to be some *predictive* processing that occurs in generating our perception [7, 8]. So perception itself is a *predicted* representation of the world, not an *actual* reflection of what's there – it's a hallucination of sorts. According to *Predictive Processing* (PP) models [7], our brain generates a prediction to represent what's likely to be causing our current sensations. So, this is more like a predictive template or model that is superimposed onto the world – a best guess about what would need to be present *out there* (in the external world) in order to 'fit' with what's happening *in here* (in my internal world of sensations).

In this view, our conscious experience is not built out of direct sensory information received by our brain. It is a predictive template that the brain generates itself. The brain then uses the sensory information from the world to later check whether its prediction was any good (to check for, so-called, *prediction error*). As philosophy lecturer, Sam Wilkinson and colleagues put it, "[the environment] *keeps our predictions in check; it keeps them accurate and world-directed*" [9].

So why might we have evolved a brain that perceives the world predictively, rather than processes it accurately? Could it be, as Hoffman argues, to prevent us from getting overwhelmed by too much information? Could it be to preserve energy resources? It's likely to be more energy-efficient for our brain to present us with a template or 'gist' of a situation than to process every single detail. Could it be to help us stay one step ahead of danger? If we are perceiving a threat that could be about to happen, then we may be more ready to deal with the threat if it does happen. Could it be to prepare or *brace* our body for protective action? Having our muscles pre-emptively braced for fight-or-flight, for example, would mean that if we did need to use fight-or-flight, our body would already be warmed up and ready to go. A system that works predictively would of course lead to 'false alarms' (what in the earlier doodle on page 10 I called 'Type I errors' or 'false positives'). However, in an evolutionary sense, this is an error that's probably worthwhile for the increased benefits to survival. Going back to our caveman ('round the camp-fire') scene at the beginning of the chapter, it is probably the ancestors who made a lot of Type I errors who passed their genes on to us.

I must point out that I am no expert in cognitive neuroscience, and my understanding of the perceptual and neural mechanisms involved is quite basic. However, I have worked for two decades (as a therapist and a scientist/researcher) with people who frequently experience perceptual hallucinations. These are people who hear voices and perceive sounds, smells, and visions of things that do not exist *out there* in the external world. They often sense a presence of someone or something that's not (physically) present. Their brains are constructing these perceptions. But why? There is no sensory signal arriving into their brains from the outside world, and yet there is a very real perception of a sound, smell, or image in their awareness. In my view, one of the biggest and most devastating errors we have made in our modern civilisations is to dismiss these kinds of experiences as pathology. We typically label these hallucinations in terms of illness, mis-firing neurons, as manifestations of a mental disorder or malfunction. But what if, one day, we were to learn that *all* perception is hallucinated?

It may be that in the future (perhaps a not-too-distant future, the way our modern cognitive neurosciences are progressing), we discover that perception is itself a form of 'controlled hallucination' [10]. And this is not a disorder or malfunction. To the contrary, this is the whole point of perception, and why evolution has given it to us – to help us to survive and navigate through our environments. To do this effectively, our brain has evolved a system that generates predictions and conjures up 'best guesses' to guide our actions. If we had *this* kind of understanding, would we be so quick to pathologise one person's perception, such as voice-hearing, just because it doesn't correspond to our own? Or would we be more inclined to ask *why*? Why is this person's brain predicting the presence of a voice? How does a voice-hearing prediction 'fit' with the current sensory signals in this person's body? Or how does a voice-hearing prediction 'fit' with the (protective) survival goals of this person?

I have recently published, with my colleague Tobyn Bell, an article that outlines a *Predictive Processing* (PP) account of voice-hearing [11], and this is a topic that we will also return to briefly at the end of Chapter 5, in the section 'remote detonators', when we explore the possible protective functions of hearing a critical voice.

For now, the important thing for us to recognise is that perceptual hallucinations are not just things that happen for those of us who come to the attention of mental health services. They can be experienced by all of us, on a continuum throughout the population [12]. Remember, we were experiencing a version of this ourselves a couple of sections back when we were hallucinating sloped lines that were in fact parallel. Another version of this is with our experience of phantom limbs and rubber hands.

Phantom limbs and rubber hands

The *phantom limb* phenomenon refers to a perception of continuing to have a limb after amputation – i.e. after this limb has been removed. Amputees will continue to perceive the presence of their phantom limb, complete with sensations such as tingles, itches, and pains [13]. Again, as with voice-hearing, these are not sensory signals arriving at our brain from an external or peripheral source. This is a hallucinated presence of signals; signals generated by the brain's own perceptual system. The *rubber hand* illusion is a well-known demonstration of body-ownership hallucination. A person is invited to sit down at a table where they can see a fake rubber hand in front of them, while their own hand is hidden from view. When they see this rubber hand being stroked with a brush, while their own (hidden) hand is simultaneously stroked, the brain mistakenly perceives the fake hand as their own. This is a neat demonstration of how visual perception is constructed from multiple other signals beyond just the visual signals that are arriving in through the eyes.

To summarise, what have we learnt so far about our brain?

Let's just briefly summarise and tie together a few different strands. So far in this chapter, we have learnt about how our brain has evolved with a strong bias towards threat. Its tagline is 'better safe than sorry'. Secondly, we have learnt that our brain is in the business of actively constructing and shaping our perceptual realities. Reality itself does play a role, but more as a secondary reference-checker than a primary *driver* of our actions. The real driving force comes from our underlying motivations, body sensations, emotions, fears, and needs. These are what shape our predictions, perceptions, and ultimately our actions. When we put these things together, we start to build a picture of a brain that: (i) is quite inclined to influence our perception and behaviour *in line with* its own goals, such as protection, which often are not even conscious to us; that (ii) doesn't particularly obey our rules of reason and logic; and that (iii) doesn't particularly prioritise the things that might be a priority to us, such as accuracy, such as happiness, such as positive mental health. Sometimes our brain's goals are directly at odds with our personal goals. And it's from this understanding and launchpad that we are now ready to jump straight into our explorative journey of controlled explosions.

Controlled explosions as a protective strategy

Controlled explosions are strategies used by our brains to protect us. Our brains create self-generated sabotage, harms, threats, and problems to avert some other greater (predicted) harm from occurring. For example, we may self-sabotage to avoid taking an action that could lead to feared consequences. We might self-criticise or self-attack to prepare or brace ourselves for the possibility of being criticised or attacked by someone else. We might self-harm to avoid or numb ourselves from painful feelings that we fear we might not be able to control. To help us identify and map out the protective functions of our controlled explosions, we are going to use a basic template that breaks this down into its two key aspects:

HARM CREATED: ....

HARM AVERTED: ....

The first aspect – harm created – involves identifying the self-inflicted harm or problem that is being created by the strategy. The second bit – harm averted – involves identifying the other (greater) predicted harm that is being avoided: the feared outcome that the controlled explosion strategy is desperately attempting to avoid.

Each of these two aspects can be mapped out using a simple visual template. This diagram visually represents how the controlled explosion comes along to divert the course *away from* the feared direction of travel. Hence, the controlled explosion is serving a protective function – it is creating a 'new' harm in order to avert a predicted (worse) harm.

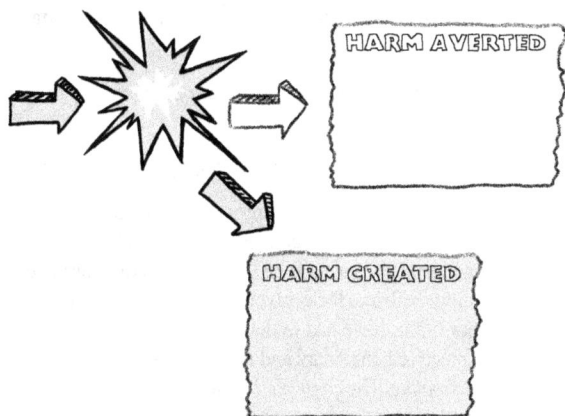

Visual template for mapping a controlled explosion

Our controlled explosions map in action

As we will be using this same two-part template throughout this book, let's get ourselves a bit more familiar with it now, with a few examples of controlled explosions in action. These examples will span across a few different domains to give us a sense of the broad range of application for this metaphor and model. We will start with some examples of how this template can be applied to common emotional struggles that we encounter in day-to-day life.

Example 1 – I am struggling with procrastination

HARM CREATED: *I keep procrastinating and putting off the very important task*

HARM AVERTED: *The shame I would feel if I failed at something important to me*

Example 2 – I am struggling with shame and indecision around food and eating

HARM CREATED: *I eat all the doughnuts and beat myself up to get it over and done with*

HARM AVERTED: *Indefinite rumination, uncertainty, and anxious tension*

Example 3 – I am struggling with anger

HARM CREATED: *I start an argument to provide a 'home' to discharge my anger*

HARM AVERTED: *The discomfort of sitting with angry feelings in my body*

Example 4 – I am struggling with anxiety and stress following a bereavement

> **HARM CREATED:** *I create dramas and chaos in my life that demand my attention*

> **HARM AVERTED:** *The painful acceptance and feelings of sadness and loss*

The controlled explosions in these examples have a personal (protective) function, in that they protect me from experiencing my own uncomfortable feelings (namely shame, anger, anxiety, and sadness). Other types of controlled explosion, however, might be more built into the evolved protective architecture of our brains. As we have seen, our brains have had to develop ways of effectively and rapidly switching on our protective behaviours and responses, such as *fight-and-flight*, as well as *submit* and *dissociate*. The *controlled explosions* metaphor is a useful parallel for understanding these processes, particularly to make sense of how our brain has developed ways to self-stimulate these responses in the interests of survival.

Example 5 – I am self-criticising and beating myself up

> **HARM CREATED:** *My self-attacking is triggering me to feel inferior, weak, small*

> **HARM AVERTED:** *The likelihood of being harmed by other people in the external world*

This self-stimulation of protective action is something I have written about extensively in an earlier book, co-authored with Eleanor Longden, in relation to voice-hearing experiences [14], but is also equally relevant to self-attacking forms of self-criticism. It might be helpful to think of this as the brain playing out both roles of a threat relationship; both the threat-*giving* and threat-*receiving* roles. The critical, attacking part (or voice) is the *giver* of threat, and on the *receiving* side of this threat, a protective action is being elicited.

With the *controlled explosions* metaphor, it is possible hold two contradictory truths in mind when it comes to self-critical parts – that yes, on one hand these are *'inner attackers'* (harmful to us) and at the same time they are also *'inner dissociation-makers'* or *'inner submission-makers'* (protecting us from harm). Often the more forceful and violent they are, the more they harm us, but also the more effective they are at switching on our protective action.

The five examples we have looked at so far have all been linked to psychological and emotional processes. However, the controlled explosion metaphor can extend to other physical and biological processes, and to medical interventions, such as understanding how a vaccination works. These examples are provided here, along with another doodle to help illustrate.

Example 6 – How a vaccine works

> **HARM CREATED:** *Add virus or antigen to mimic infection and to prime immune response*

HARM AVERTED: *Having a body that is unprepared to recognise and fight a disease*

Example 7 – When our body is fighting a virus (like Covid-19)

HARM CREATED: *Raise temperature and send to bed with sweats, chills and dizziness*

HARM AVERTED: *Virus spreading and infecting multiple cells throughout the body*

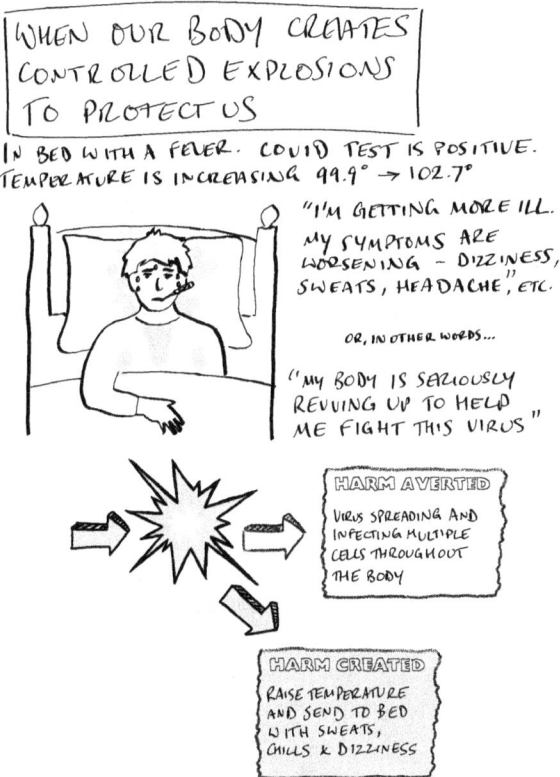

DOODLE: "When our body creates controlled explosions to protect us"

Meet the bomb squad

In this book, the bomb squad are the characters responsible for creating controlled explosions. The bomb squad is comprised of three units: the Self-Sabotage Unit, the Self-Criticism Unit, and the Self-Harm Unit. Each of these units creates slightly different types of controlled explosion, and each member has a slightly different focus and objective for how they go about their work.

There are five members per unit, each with a unique name (such as **PRO-CRASTINATOR**, **DISSOCIATOR**, and **CHAOS-CREATOR**) to help us keep track of the various functions of the controlled explosions.

The following diagrams will orientate you to all the bomb squad units and members, as well as to their headquarters, and the equipment they keep in their kit room to support their controlled explosions ('containment vessels', 'disrupters', and 'remote detonators'). The second flow diagram (page 25) includes a summary of all the different members, their objectives, and what their equipment is used for. This also serves the purpose of providing a map of the overall book structure, with each chapter and section introducing these in turn.

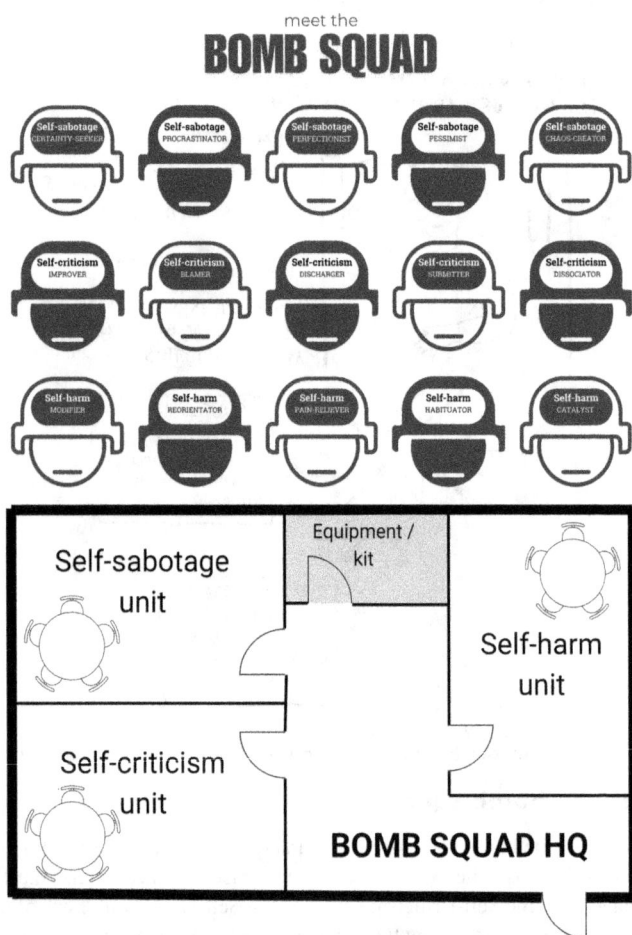

The bomb squad and their headquarters

The Bomb Squad

(Mission: To protect us by creating controlled explosions)

Self-Sabotage Unit	**Self-Criticism Unit**	**Self-Harm Unit**
(Controlled explosions that can derail our lives and plans)	(Controlled explosions that can harm us psychologically)	(Controlled explosions that can harm us physically)
CERTAINTY-SEEKER – to create an affirmed self and a predictable world	**IMPROVER** – to create a self-improvement response	**MODIFIER** – to create improvement by body modifications
PROCRASTINATOR – to create distractions, temptations and delays	**BLAMER** – to create a feeling of agency and control	**REORIENTATOR** – to create diversions and reorientation
PERFECTIONIST – to create exceptional standards and error-checks	**DISCHARGER** – to discharge and complete a fight/flight response	**PAIN-RELIEVER** – to elicit natural pain relief and numbing
PESSIMIST – to create low expectations and anticipate problems	**SUBMITTER** – to create a submissive response	**HABITUATOR** – to create desentitisation, habituation and mastery
CHAOS-CREATOR – to create drama, chaos and catastrophe	**DISSOCIATOR** – to create a dissociative response	**CATALYST** – to amplify, speed up and complete a response

Equipment / Kit

(Equipment used to support controlled explosions)

CONTAINMENT VESSELS – to hold and contain emotional activation	**DISRUPTERS** – to disrupt processes that could lead to harm	**REMOTE DETONATORS** – to initiate impact from an external location

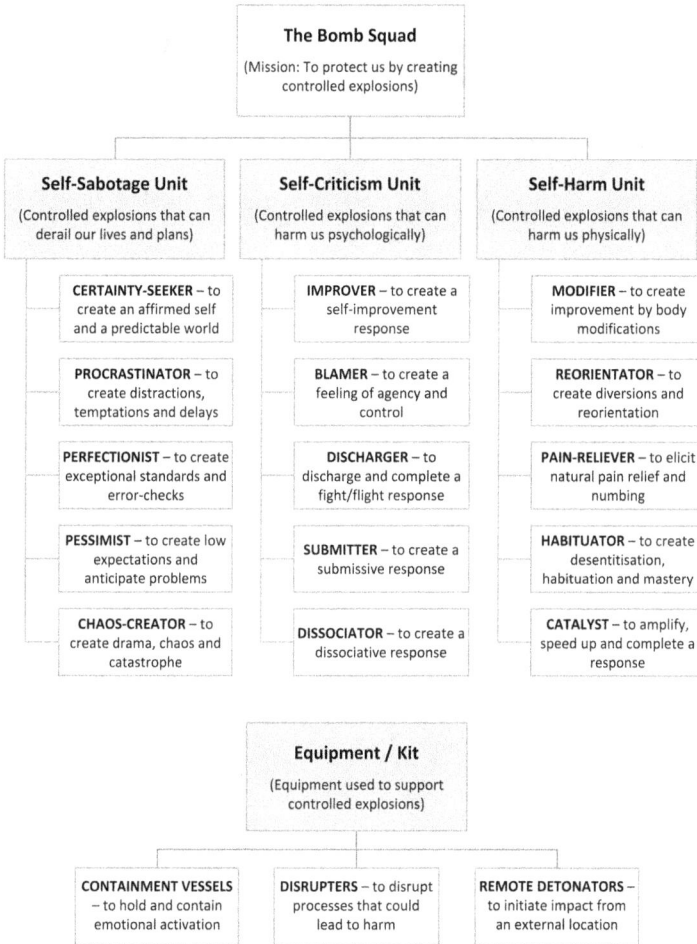

The bomb squad units, members, with their objectives and equipment

Note

1 You will notice that there are a few hand-drawn 'doodles' dotted throughout this book. I have decided to keep some of my figures and tables in their original, hand-drafted, form because it feels more personal that way. There are other digitally built figures too (more professional-looking!) but I just wanted to keep a handful of doodles in here too to give you a more personal sense of the sketching and working on ideas that went into developing this book.

Part II

Controlled explosions

The bomb squad

Chapter 2

Self-Sabotage Unit

Controlled explosions that can derail our lives and plans

Chapter summary

This chapter explores examples of self-sabotage, particularly focusing on the familiar patterns of things like procrastination, which most of us can relate to in our day-to-day life, as well as perfectionism, which can really sabotage our progress and direction forward. The Self-Sabotage Unit typically create the kinds of controlled explosions that derail our lives and plans. Procrastination, for example, can derail us by diverting our minds towards distractions, temptations, and chaos. Perfectionism can derail us by creating impossible standards and rules that we can never achieve. This chapter explores some possible functions of these inner saboteurs and considers important questions about what might be some of the bigger harms that are being avoided or prevented.

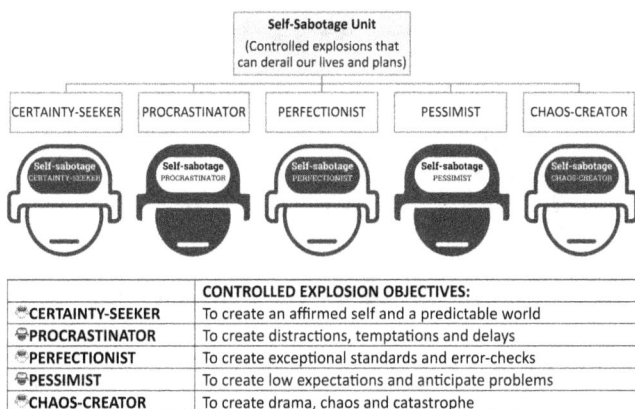

Self-Sabotage Unit
(Controlled explosions that can derail our lives and plans)

| CERTAINTY-SEEKER | PROCRASTINATOR | PERFECTIONIST | PESSIMIST | CHAOS-CREATOR |

	CONTROLLED EXPLOSION OBJECTIVES:
CERTAINTY-SEEKER	To create an affirmed self and a predictable world
PROCRASTINATOR	To create distractions, temptations and delays
PERFECTIONIST	To create exceptional standards and error-checks
PESSIMIST	To create low expectations and anticipate problems
CHAOS-CREATOR	To create drama, chaos and catastrophe

Members, roles, and objectives of the Self-Sabotage Unit

DOI: 10.4324/9781003559924-5

The term *self-sabotage* is typically used to describe situations when we create barriers towards our own goals. There are a number of ways that we do this, so within the bomb squad, this has a special unit of its own. Let's now meet the unit members one-by-one.

CERTAINTY-SEEKER: to create an affirmed self and a predictable world

Above all else, our brains crave predictability. Experiencing familiarity and certainty in the world means that we can predict the future. And being able to predict and anticipate what is about to happen next is key to our survival. As it happens, our brains have even evolved a system for rewarding our ability to predict the future. As neuroscientist Beau Lotto says, it releases *"feel-good"* chemicals into our body when our predictions are confirmed, and it activates stress emotions when our predictions are challenged [5]. To fulfil our certainty-seeking impulses and cravings, we tend to look for familiar patterns in the world. This is largely to do with survival – recognising patterns allows anticipation of what is to come, so we can also stay one step ahead of danger. But it is also to do with efficiency – looking for patterns allows us to process information more efficiently, and by using fewer energy resources.

An important job of our **CERTAINTY-SEEKER** is to ensure that our world is perceived as an orderly place, ruled by predictable patterns of cause-and-effect. Sustaining this perception is adaptive – it helps us to function and navigate our environment with some degree of confidence. It would be extremely hard to tolerate an uncertain world, where cause-and-effect patterns were random, predictions were futile, and where experiences of good and bad things happening to us (such as rewards and punishments) were doled out in a haphazard way [15]. In such an existence, we would likely be, at best, perpetually stressed and disoriented, and at worst, despairing, hopeless, and paralysed.

So, experiencing certainty helps us to function and feel in control. It makes us feel great with its natural, built-in dopamine hit. It's an efficient use of our limited energy resources for processing the world, and it brings a survival advantage to our species. So, what's not to like? Well, as with most things to do with this evolved (*tricky*) brain of ours, there is a trade-off.

Connecting patterns and causes in unrelated events

The many benefits of certainty-seeking unfortunately come with a cost. Firstly, it creates blind spots and inaccuracies in how we perceive the world. Our tendency to look for familiar patterns in the world, rather than looking directly at the reality of what is there, of course produces perceptual biases and errors (see earlier section on *Predictive Processing*, page 17). Other biases occur through our reasoning and cognitions, i.e. how we think about the world, make sense of it, and attribute cause-and-effect. For example, our certainty-seeking brain has a strong confirmation bias [16], in that it prioritises information which fits with or confirms our own beliefs or expectations, while deprioritising that which is disconfirmatory. Our brain also has a tendency to make connections between events that are, in fact, unrelated.

A predictable world is one that has fairness and justice; where things happen *for a reason* – i.e. rewards come when rewards are due or deserved, and punishments come when punishments are due or deserved (see Just World Theory from the social psychologist, Melvin Lerner [17]). In striving for this predictable world, our **CERTAINTY-SEEKER** will sometimes infer a cause to something that is random or infer an overly simple cause to something with complex and multiple causes. This can involve, for example, attributing the cause of an event to some of our own personal actions or traits. This is called a self-affirming bias [18]. This can feel great when there are good things happening to us – it can really boost our confidence and self-esteem (*'it was all my hard work that opened up this new career opportunity'* or *'that was excellent judgement of mine to bet on that winning horse!'*) Where this becomes more problematic, however, is when bad things are happening.

Unfortunately, but inevitably, negative experiences will happen in our lives. And for some of us, tragically, but through no fault of our own, there can be a pile up of many bad things happening in different aspects of our life, or repeatedly in the same aspect. Even though these events may be completely random and out of our personal control, our internal **CERTAINTY-SEEKER** can often still make this about us. The likelihood is that it will be searching desperately for a cause – to pin the blame on *someone* or *something*. For example, when we experience the death of a loved one, we might find ourselves feeling guilty (*"it's my fault"*) or angry (*"it's that person over there's fault"*), and maybe switching between the two, as if we were grappling for some causal explanation to attach meaning – and thus satisfy our need for certainty.

Remember, the **CERTAINTY-SEEKER** is on a protective mission to avoid the danger of uncertainty at all costs. It cares more about averting this (potentially greater) harm, than any costs around 'accuracy' (i.e. attributing an incorrect cause) or indeed 'mental health' (i.e. guilt or shame in attributing a cause to self, and maybe even self-punishment). The tendency to allocate blame to oneself, as opposed to an external event, is likely to increase in relation to the greater frequency of adverse events. (Also see the **BLAMER** section later). For example, if someone's home is robbed multiple times, they are more likely to start wondering, for example, *"Am I being targeted? And if so, why? Is it someone I've upset? Is it something I've done?"* Even if there are bad things happening across multiple different and unrelated areas of my life, I might be tempted to conclude that perhaps this has something to do with me because I am the only connection that binds these events together – I am the common denominator.

There is a self-referencing bias in humans that can be traced back through many historical examples as well – for example, how our ancestors used to attribute natural phenomena like the weather (such as flooding or drought) to the will of the Gods, perhaps as a punishment from the Gods. (*"Why are the Gods disapproving? We must deserve this. It must be something we have done. Quick, think of all the bad things we have done recently".*) We can even get a sense of this self-referencing bias in the more modern day and trivial context of watching a sports game on the TV. Imagine you are there watching the game. It is entering an exciting final phase, the teams are tightly poised, and you briefly leave the room to grab a drink. But when you come back in the room, you find that the other team has scored! Although of course you know that there is no logical connection between these two events, it is hard to avoid at least a fleeting sense of personal responsibility for your team's demise!

Creating inaccurate perceptions and attributions, particularly self-blaming attributions, could be one example of a controlled explosion deployed by the **CERTAINTY-SEEKER**. However, this is only the beginning of how far it is prepared to go to achieve the goal of certainty for us. Such is its determination that it will even manipulate our behaviour to create a future situation in which the reality of the world falls into line with the (inaccurate) predictions we have made! Psychologists have long been familiar with the concept of *self-fulfilling prophecy* [19], where our predictions and expectations actually become re-alities. This can have either positive or negative outcomes (depending on the prediction), but in the spirit of *controlled explosions*, we will be particularly focusing on examples of when this can have a negative outcome – when a prediction leads to a prediction-fulfilling behaviour that is self-defeating.

Engineering a situation to 'fit' my prediction

In this section, we will consider some examples where we might find our-selves engaging in self-sabotaging actions in service of avoiding uncertainty. This could be sabotaging anything from our daily tasks, projects, and goals to our careers, relationships, and general well-being. By exploring these in this book, my hope is that you may be able to start noticing if and when this may be happening in your life. Our ability to notice this, to understand why (and that it's a normal, natural part of being human, and not our fault) will empower us to make choices. For example, we may be able to choose between *"do I continue to accept that I am sabotaging this goal or opportunity for the sake of certainty?"* or *"do I want to address this by tolerating a bit of uncer-tainty here to see what will come of this?"*

The first example for us to consider is that of a student who strongly be-lieves they are not good at a subject and that they will fail their end-of-year exam. The student predicts exam failure, and they subsequently engage in ac-tions (such as not putting much effort into studying and revising) that greatly increase the chances that their predicted outcome will come true. Making this prediction in the first place may itself be a type of controlled explosion designed to avoid the anticipated pain they would feel if they had set a higher expectation and failed (which we return to when we meet another member of the Self-Sabotage Unit, the **PESSIMIST**). But regardless of where this prediction has come from, or how accurate it is, we can see how the student's subsequent actions are actively creating a new reality that serves the initial prediction in a self-defeating way. The prediction has become a self-fulfilling prophecy. This can happen in many areas of life – if we think we are not very good at something, we may not try our best and then end up performing worse than we would have had we made a different prediction.

Importantly, it's not just our own predictions about ourselves that can shape our behaviours and influence our future realities; it's also other people's expectations of us. A number of studies have shown, for example, that a teacher's expectations of their students can shape the students' performances [20]. Social stereotypes are also thought to work via this same mechanism, whereby the expectations of a group or subgroup (categorised, for example, by their shared race, gender, or social class) can influence and shape that group's behaviour in line with these social expectations [21].

The **CERTAINTY-SEEKER** likes us to have a fixed sense of our identity – to know who we are, and to know who our 'people' are. This identity fixing is self-affirming and gives us sense of self integrity and belonging. However, the cost is that it comes with strong predictions and self-fulfilling prophecies – *"I am good at this and bad at that"* – which can be both self-affirming and self-defeating. Pioneering psychologist, Carol Dweck, has done some wonderful work highlighting the costs of having a "fixed mindset", especially among students in education, and her term "growth mindset" [22] has become a key principle and mantra for many in the education sector.

In social psychology studies, it has been demonstrated that similar processes can play out in our relationships. If participants are led to believe (falsely) that another person dislikes them, they will sit further away, engage in less eye contact, and disagree more than participants who are led to believe that the person likes them [23]. Another well-known example of self-fulfilling prophecy is in the economy and financial markets, where studies have shown that speculative predictions of economic change can impact people's financial decisions and behaviours before these changes are realised [24]. Again, an expectation influences a behaviour, which brings the future reality into line with the prediction. And again, this could be positive or negative. In the 2008 financial crisis, there were reports of *bank runs*, where customers predicted a bank would collapse, and so rushed to withdraw all their money, which of course led to the collapse of the bank.

The predictions and attributions we make (to avoid feelings of uncertainty) could turn out to be costly and harmful. Strong, fixed, negative predictions about ourselves could result in self-defeating behaviour. Also, if we attribute ourselves to be the cause of negative events, this could result in other difficult feelings such as guilt and shame, as well as self-criticising and self-punishing behaviour (which will be explored in depth when we introduce the other two bomb squad units – the Self-Criticism and Self-Harm Units). In their conclusions from a series of studies on self-defeat, Callan, Kay, and Dawtry suggested that people engage in self-destructive behaviours not because they are primarily motivated for self-destruction, but because there is a "trade-off" between the advantages of sustaining a belief that the world is "fair, predictable, and orderly" and the disadvantages of self-defeating (self-costly) actions that sustain that belief [15]. This book is all about trade-offs. So, mapping onto our framework of *controlled explosions*, the trade-off here is that the **CERTAINTY-SEEKER** is creating a harm (a self-defeating action) that serves to avert another harm (the fear of existing in an uncertain, random, haphazard world).

> **HARM CREATED:** *I sabotage potentially anything (personal goals, career, relationships)*
>
> **HARM AVERTED:** *To avoid the experience of uncertainty*

Flirting around the edges of certainty (but not too far!)

While certainty-seeking is indeed a strong innate force within us, we also have an innate (survival) imperative to seek out novelty, to grow, learn, explore, and develop new skills. This requires us to go out of our comfort zone – to venture slightly outside, at least round the edges, of certainty. Entering uncertain territory will of course elicit stressful feelings for us, but in a recent account by Miller, White, and Scrivner, an intriguing case is made for why we might also have an attraction to these uncertain conditions. The authors base their ideas around the reasons why we are drawn to horror movies, suggesting that we experience pleasure and reward in being able to *resolve* uncertainty. Using a *Predictive Processing* framework, they argue that uncertain and volatile environments offer an ideal opportunity for experiencing resolvable prediction errors, and suggest that horror movies have the "ability to push us to that edge of our predictive capabilities" with "a 'just-right' amount of fear" [25]. This also relates to thrill-seeking sports, where we experience pleasure in pushing ourselves beyond our limits. We experience both pleasure and fear. As well as our pull towards certainty-seeking, we also have a pull towards sensation-seeking, and this can sometimes become a bit of a tussle or tug-of-war (see doodle). However, importantly, watching movies and participating in extreme sports are both choices, i.e. there is an intentional, *controlled* entry into the feelings of fear and uncertainty. We can experience the pleasure and thrill with the safety and certainty of knowing that we can stop at any time we choose. This is why we could argue that this is not quite the same as a real, genuine uncertainty (i.e. totally random, disordered, haphazard). This is more like flirting around the edges – a controlled entry into a predictable and resolvable uncertainty. We still know *how* and *when* we can return to our comfort zone, and we will have a good feeling when we come back, knowing that we have mastered this. Some of these themes will be picked up again and elaborated later when we meet another co-member of this unit, the **CHAOS-CREATOR**.

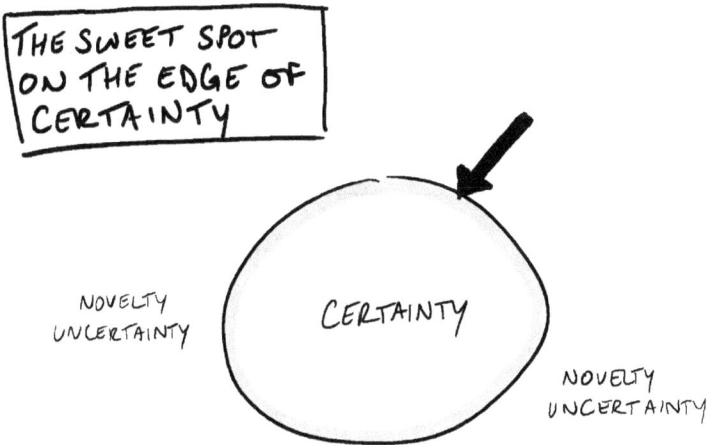

THE SWEET SPOT ON THE EDGE OF CERTAINTY

NOVELTY UNCERTAINTY

CERTAINTY

NOVELTY UNCERTAINTY

TUG OF WAR

CERTAINTY-SEEKING

SENSATION-SEEKING

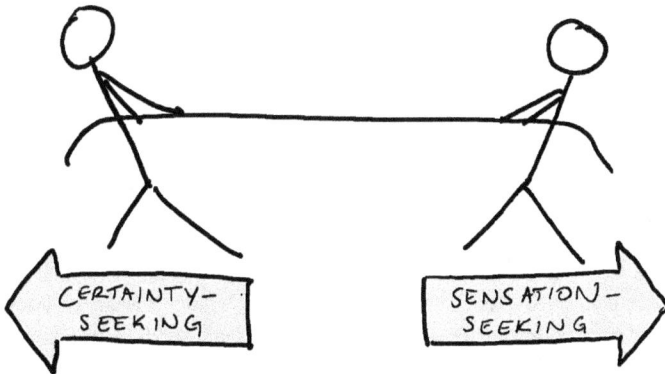

DOODLE: "The sweet spot on the edge of certainty"

PROCRASTINATOR: to create distractions, temptations, and delays

The next role to introduce in the Self-Sabotage Unit is the **PROCRASTINA-TOR**. This one is particularly relevant for me while I sit here writing a book, because this member of the bomb squad is here with me right now in full force. The main function of this member is to use delay-tactics against us. If I have set myself a period of time for book-writing, for example, my **PRO-CRASTINATOR**'s job is to fill this time with distractions.

"Hey Charlie, have you checked the sports results?"

Some of the distractions are more subtle, in that they look like they are trying to help me with my goal (writing), but actually they are delaying me from starting.

"So what do you need to have in place before you can start writing? A cup of tea? A timetable? A colour-coding system? A new laptop?"

I arrived two nights ago in a place called Glencoe on the West coast of Scotland, which is one of the most beautiful places I have ever been to. And I spent the whole morning yesterday scrolling through an app about the best walks you can do in the area. So let's just check-in with this for a minute, and look at what's going on here: I took time off specifically to write a book, and yet I chose a beauty spot with some of the most perfect ways to distract me from this task. Nice one, **PROCRASTINATOR**. But it was not finished there. I ended up choosing a walk from the app that said it was a "2 hour" route, which is quite a long walk for me, but my **PROCRASTINATOR** justi-fied this by saying:

"If you do a long walk first, then you'll feel more satisfied, and can then start writing your book in earnest without further distractions."

Good thinking, **PROCRASTINATOR**! Now it turns out that the app was wrong, and the walk actually took 4 hours, and all the way up a mountain called Pap of Glencoe. By the time I'd finished, I was shattered and starving. I had to eat a late lunch and then spend about an hour resting my legs in the bath. Now I don't think this bomb squad member was fully culpable for the entire controlled explosion (for example, I don't think it arranged it so that the app would tell me the wrong information!), but it certainly played its part. Perhaps it knows that if it does a good enough job of diverting and distracting me in the first place, then other distractions will naturally follow. I eventually got down to start some writing at about 4pm, just as it was about to get dark. Day 1: **PROCRASTINATOR** wins the day.

So, why does it do this? Remember, with *controlled explosions*, the explosion is self-generated in service of preventing some (bigger) harm. So what bigger harm is our procrastination protecting us from? On the surface, writing a book might not seem like such a harmful thing, but let's dig down into it a bit more. Firstly, there is fear of failure. Setting out on a task, particularly one that is important to us personally, is scary. What if we fail? What if it does not meet the expectations we held? Starting this task is a fearful moment because this is the moment when something transforms from just an *idea* into a *reality*. An idea is much safer, and much more exciting. With an idea, you can happily stay with the good feelings. The reality is entirely different. It involves pain, struggle, effort. And you have to come face-to-face with the very real possibility that this idea, this fantasy, may not look the same in reality as you'd imagined. The emotions involved with the idea or fantasy are possibly excitement and pleasure, whereas the emotions involved in the reality are potentially fear, shame, and sadness. It's a risk to just let that play out. Our **PROCRASTINATOR** steps in to derail that and prevent it from happening. All the timetabling, scheduling, reprioritising tasks. This is partly avoidance, but also partly to exert control over the exact timing of feeling the pain. Remember, the Bermondsey bomb explosion was timed for precisely 9am on a specific day in March. Avoid ..., delay ..., avoid ..., delay ..., until *the perfect moment* for a prepared and controlled exposure to the painful emotions.

Completing little tasks gives you little positive feelings

The **PROCRASTINATOR** is not only helping us to avoid uncomfortable feelings. There are also a number of short-term rewards and rewarding feelings to be had, to which this bomb squad member is also quite attracted. The mini-achievements and rewards I experience, for example, from seeing that I got a 'like' on social media or from buying something with 'one click' in an online store. Adding rewarding feelings is not just about overriding a negative feeling, it has an allure of its own. In fact, our brains are programmed to need it and to seek it out.

We evolved in environments of scarcity, so it was very important for our brains to develop a reward-seeking motivational system to keep driving us to seek out new experiences. We are prepared to venture into uncertainty because we know that we will be rewarded if we are able to develop mastery over the uncertainty. Uncertainty is uncomfortable, so there has to be some kind of reward that comes from it. The rewards are feelings of power and mastery. Having an experience of mastering the unknown leaves you feeling powerful – this is because you are newly discovering some abilities in yourself that you didn't previously realise you had. Some of the rewards are learnt, for example, the rewards you got from your parents when you achieved difficult tasks in childhood (learning to walk, ride a bicycle, and so on).

Other rewards may be more intrinsic, for example, the experience of feeling your own progression in yourself. Uncertainty also opens up the opportunity for having creative insights (a new angle – similar to how a metaphor opens up a new framework in which to perceive things).

> *In an emotional state, people may notice stimuli in the environment that they would usually overlook, or they may interpret stimuli in novel ways because of their emotional perspective.*
>
> Lubert & Getz, citing Isen, 1987 [26])

Interestingly, a lot of people assume that the neurotransmitter dopamine is released when our brain receives a reward, but actually it is released in the anticipation – i.e. in the excitement and craving period, where there is still some uncertainty of whether or not there will be a reward. The anticipatory cravings are likely to be stronger if (a) we have previously learnt that rewards may come in this situation (i.e. there is an expectation), but also if (b) the uncertain period of 'no reward yet' is extended. In this tantalising space, we are braced for either maybe a reward will come or maybe it won't. The longer we spend here – the more we are tantalisingly close to a reward – the more our senses are heightened. Our body is alive with tingling, buzzy feelings. We might feel an urge for movement, twitching, rocking, pacing. If we do manage to stay seated, perhaps we find ourselves poised – braced 'on the edge of our seat' while the internal energy and sensations bubble up inside our body. The body is preparing us for something – it could be reward. Maybe. Maybe not.

The most exciting sports games are the ones that are too close to call. For example, in team-sports the scoreboard lead might switch multiple times between opponents, or the game is so evenly matched that it has to go into extra time. These are what the sports journalists call 'thrillers'. The excitement is in uncertainty itself, not in the resolution of the uncertainty. The thrill builds as uncertainty increases, not decreases.

In *Predictive Processing* terms, the gap is widening between prediction and outcome. So the chance of a positive prediction error (it's too close to predict, and then we win!) increases. So dopamine favours unpredictable reward over predictable reward.

The **PROCRASTINATOR** knows this. Writing a book all the way through to completion will be a reward – no doubt. But this is a very slow-burning predictable reward. When I finish this book, I won't have buzzy, excited feelings. I won't be braced on the edge of my seat. Well, at least not in relation to the book-finishing experience. If anything, the thrill will now come from the new task that is unlocked – the submission, publication, and opening the book up to the world and the highly uncertain judgements and reactions of the general public. *"Will they or won't they approve?" "What* *star rating will they give on the website?"* At that point I will now be bracing myself for the uncertainty of success or failure. Maybe joy, contentment, and pride. Maybe disappointment, humiliation, and shame. Three years of my life wasted? Or not?

Going to Fiji tomorrow (Bear Grylls)

I have recently been reading a book with my youngest son before bedtime, called *A Survival Guide for Life* by Bear Grylls, where one of the tips for becoming highly productive with to-do lists and tasks is to put ourselves under the pressure of a deadline. The context is of a man who was travelling to Fiji tomorrow at quite short notice and suddenly becomes hyper-focused and efficient in getting through his tasks – getting everything ticked-off and finished before the trip; hence the idea, *"imagine if I had to go to Fiji every day!"* [27]. How productive would we be if we could re-create that 'Fiji' attitude or mindset in our daily lives? And how far would we go to create this 'pressured', but productive, mindset for ourselves?

Many of us recognise that we do work better under a healthy dose of pressure and stress. A deadline can certainly focus and sharpen our minds. When revising for an exam, many of us leave revision till the final week or so before. Generally, the motivation here is to do better (so not necessarily a self-sabotage), but there can be quite a fine line between self-motivating and self-sabotaging. It can be a risky business bringing self-inflicted pressure into our own lives. In a way, we are trying to (intentionally) create an uncertain 'thrill' state for our brains to thrive *("will I or won't I get my revision done"*; *"will I or won't I get through my to-do list"*). It's a controlled entry into a state of panic to switch on our alertness – intentionally sabotaging ourselves to get the best out of us. *"I'll leave it till the very last minute and do it then."* The motivation here is complex, because I am intentionally neglecting to do this thing now, with the intention that my neglect will result in heightened urgency of attention to it later! But what if the 'later' point arrives and something even more urgent comes up?

The classic one for me is before my break for the Christmas holidays. I set all my work deadlines for the week before Christmas, because I know that every year I will take one or two weeks off. It's the only consistently regular time off for me. So there I am, the week before Christmas with suddenly a mountain of all the built-up tasks I've been procrastinating. Four deadlines in four days. The intention was that somehow in that week before Christmas I would be able to summon up my inner superhero. In my imagination, I would be there in full 'Fiji' mode, knocking out the tasks of my to-do list with a superhuman ease. This would be similar, I imagined, to how the character Neo dodges bullets in the film, *The Matrix*.

However, the reality is that there I am now gradually realising that I've piled up the four most tedious tasks – the hardest ones. I'm also suddenly remembering that Christmas is when there are a flurry of other non-work commitments, and at a rate that's far higher than any other time of the year: shopping for presents – up 400%; social invitations to drinks and parties – up 500%; emails from other people – up 1000% (while everyone else scrambles to clear their own emails and to-do lists before the Christmas break). So actually, all I've done is shifted my *most tedious* tasks to the *most impossible* time. Even Neo from *The Matrix* wouldn't be able to handle 20,000 bullets heading towards him all at once. The point here is that even in cases where there is some degree of good intention from the **PROCRASTINATOR** (an intention to help, rather than to harm), it often turns out to be harmful anyway.

The problem is it's a risky strategy. If we leave everything until the final day before Fiji, in the hope that our dopamine-inspired inner super-human self will come to our rescue, the problem is it might not. We might have created a prediction *"ooh how exciting, maybe I won't be able to get it done"* and then we don't. The prediction comes true. As we will see later when we meet the **PESSIMIST**, often our predictions become self-fulfilling prophecies. Making a prediction that I won't succeed is a bit like playing with fire. On the one hand, this 'failure' prediction could set up an opportunity for a prediction error that awakens our inner superhuman. But on the other hand, this 'failure' prediction could greatly increase the chances of failure. How do we find the *sweet spot* in the middle?

We need to have just enough uncertainty to awaken and energise us, and yet just enough certainty to make sure that we don't fail or give up. Maybe that's the trick here: rather than predicting failure, can we simultaneously hold two competing predictions – the *"maybe I will, maybe I won't"* state. The *"will I, won't I"*. Both–and, rather than either–or.

This is the sports game equivalent of being in extra time, as the clock ticks down, after seeing the teams exchange the lead back-and-forth throughout. For the viewer, there are two equally strong predictive models for the outcome. If I was a sports coach or sports psychologist, I might be coaching the players in how to not overly predict winning or defeat – to stay in the flow of excitement of not-knowing, to ride the wave of uncertainty. If you are *too* attached to your prediction of winning, you might get complacent, and the heightening of your senses might fade down a little. If you are *too* attached to your prediction of losing, your actions might align to the predictive model, and new information to the contrary might be prevented from being perceived. Can you straddle both? Are you able to hold a predictive paradox in your perception – maybe this is where you can feel most alive.

Of course, the coaching advice would be different depending on the historical context, or the run-of-form of that team. So, for the team that are used to losing, I might try and help them to build up their winning prediction so that the winning and losing models carry similar weight. For the team that are used to winning, I might try to help them building up their losing model so that the two models can coexist with a similar strength.

Back to the 'tug-of-war' between certainty-seeking and sensation-seeking

So when it comes to procrastination, it is helpful to remember that the lure away from the task (the email, spreadsheet, or book you're working on) is not necessarily to do with the rewards you can receive elsewhere. It may be more to do with the brain wanting to switch gear, from a slow-burning feeling of predictable monotony to a feeling of unpredictable novelty. The anticipatory state of being uncertain about whether or not there will be rewards. Your brain might be seeking the energising thrill of novelty. Away from the mundane monotony of the task and into the exciting unknown. Away from the predictability into the dopamine thrill of not knowing what will happen next. The little smartphone sitting next to me on the desk offers me a treasure trove of 'the unknown'. If I opened my Instagram feed right now, I could be immediately immersed in a rapid sequence of about 20 unknown, diverse experiences in the space of only one or two minutes. My brain craves novelty and uncertainty. The addictive part of social media may not just be in the receiving of 'likes', but more in the anticipatory not knowing of whether or not I will receive a 'like'.

> **HARM CREATED:** *I neglect a task by seeking a novel experience/ sensation*
>
> **HARM AVERTED:** *To avoid the experience of task monotony*

The harm created by the **PROCRASTINATOR** is often in the form of neglect – as in the neglect, desertion, and abandonment of a specific task, goal, or duty. The degree of harm is of course highly dependent on the nature of what is being neglected. The word 'harm' might feel far too strong for some of the day-to-day versions of procrastination, such as scrolling social media to avoid the effort of hanging up that picture that's been leaning against the wall for three months. But at the other end of the scale, 'harm' would be a very appropriate way to describe, for example, the neglect of a child through avoiding tasks linked to their care, health, and basic needs. In the middle, there may be other forms of neglect that could feel fairly minor and insignificant in the moment, but could become more harmful over time. For example, neglecting to pay your bills, or putting off changing that battery in the smoke alarm.

The **PROCRASTINATOR** seeks novelty to avoid monotony. But the problem is that many of life's important and essential tasks *are* incredibly monotonous and repetitive. If you have a child, they generally need to be fed three times a day. Every day. They need to be clothed. Every day. This is highly repetitive. Self-care can be very repetitive too. Brushing your teeth. Exercising. Sleeping. All pretty boring, mundane, repetitive acts. For many of us, the **PROCRASTINATOR**'s novelty-seeking, sensation-seeking efforts can lead to sabotaging and neglecting these essential parts of our self-care and well-being.

PERFECTIONIST: to create exceptional standards and error checks

Another role in the Self-Sabotage Unit is the **PERFECTIONIST**. Like the **PROCRASTINATOR**, a lot of the **PERFECTIONIST**'s work functions to support avoidance of things that are difficult and uncomfortable, and to avoid the fear of failure. However, while the **PROCRASTINATOR** often switches our attention to other tasks, the **PERFECTIONIST** typically stays 'on task', but with a hyper-focus and attention to detail with the hope of ensuring that errors are not being made.

The **PERFECTIONIST** also distracts us from the direction we are heading by overthinking every single minor detail along the way, scanning for things that are not exactly right. So not only is it impossible to achieve the task to the correct standard, but even if it were possible, it would be very hard to make progress anyway because of all the minor details that need checking, tweaking, re-tweaking, and double checking. Often more time is spent on modifying details repeatedly than on doing the task itself. Because we always fall short of the **PERFECTIONIST**'s standards, and we struggle to make any meaningful progress on the task, the scene is perfectly set for the self-critic to enter. (We will meet the Self-Criticism Unit in the next chapter.)

It may be the case that the standard-setting is itself a subtle controlled explosion tactic. For example, when setting me a standard that is impossible to achieve, my **PERFECTIONIST** might be subtly easing my path towards avoidance: *"If I set an impossible standard for Charlie, then not only will there be constant cause for distraction, procrastination, avoidance while he's working on the project, but also, he will eventually reach a point of having to admit defeat, and abandon it altogether."*

HARM CREATED: *I am rigorously error-checking against an impossible standard*

HARM AVERTED: *Fear of making an error, failure, and possibly criticism/punishment*

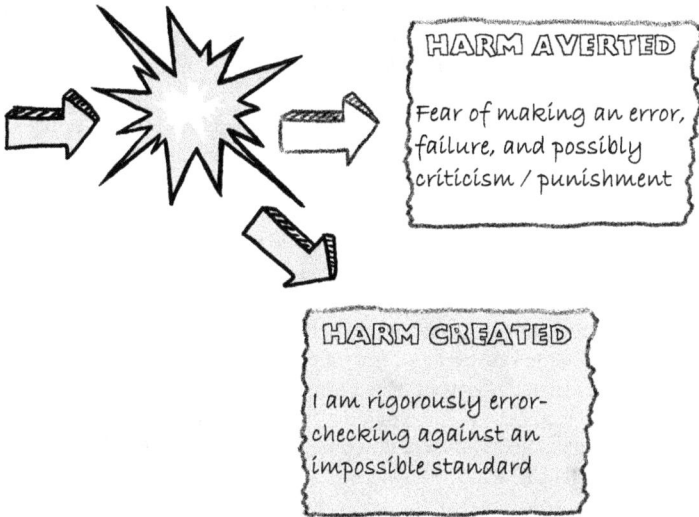

HARM AVERTED

Fear of making an error, failure, and possibly criticism / punishment

HARM CREATED

I am rigorously error-checking against an impossible standard

Perfectionism

The primary motivation is often to avoid failure. Our **PERFECTIONIST** is trying to help us avoid failure by error-checking, but the standard it is using to error-check against is often an impossible standard – hence, why it gets caught in an unresolvable loop. It is futile. Error-checking in itself is a very good thing. Having high standards itself is a good thing. But of course, the trade-off is that high standards open the door wider to underperforming. And then both high standards and underperforming fuel error-checking.

HIGH STANDARDS ↔ UNDER PERFORMING

With perfectionism, some people see this as a good trait (for instance something they will readily mention at a job interview to impress the potential employer), but other people really struggle with this, and the suffering this causes. Interestingly, in job interviews, I have noticed that when a question comes up asking a candidate to name their strengths and weaknesses, they will often say "*I'm a perfectionist*" as a weakness, although secretly hoping their interviewer sees that as a strength in disguise! In this book, we are exploring the side of perfectionism that is self-sabotaging, in that it causes problems for us.

The self-critic, who we will meet in the next chapter, can add further weight to the avoidance by making us feel demotivated and depressed. The more we get demotivated, the more the **PERFECTIONIST** demands of us as an attempt to re-boost our self-esteem. But the consequence is that we often end up with multiple uncompleted projects, and hence more ammunition for the self-critic. The self-critical ruminations and loops potentially have the additional knock-on effect of disrupting and diminishing some of the key resources we rely on to deal with tasks and challenges, such as our sleep, health, and relationships.

So what is the **PERFECTIONIST** helping us avoid and protecting us from? We have already considered the fear of failure, and coupled with this, might also be a fear of judgement. Perfectionism might also have a flavour of procrastination about it, in terms of avoidance of the uncomfortable feelings involved in doing tasks. If I am supposed to be writing a book, but all I'm doing is spending all day adjusting the margins and changing the font, is this perfectionism or procrastination? Probably a bit of both. Mental focus and exertion *are* tiring. Tasks requiring problem-solving *are* stressful. Moving forward with the next aspect of a task might feel more draining (in the moment) than tweaking aspects of the task that have already been done. A little tweak of a previous aspect can provide a 'quick win' and reward or gratification for minimal effort (similar to the quick gratification that is enjoyed by the **PROCRASTINATOR** who aborts a task in order to check their social media for 'likes').

The world is only too ready to feed our need to distract. The combination of our Self-Sabotaging Unit's desire to avoid uncomfortable feelings, along with society's desire to grab our attention and give us quick hits, is a very tricky combination indeed.

"Hey Charlie, would you rather struggle on with this task of writing a book (which at best will give you delayed reward, in about three years, or at worst will give you no reward at all) or would you prefer to watch this reel?"

Rock climbing: tinkering with safety gear or enjoying view?

One of my favourite metaphors is rock climbing. This has been massively inspired by my friend and colleague Kate Lucre, who herself is a keen climber, as she has written about in her excellent book, *Compassion Focused Group Psychotherapy* [28]. When we are engaged with a difficult task, it can sometimes be helpful to bring a metaphor like this to mind. *"Am I enjoying this climb or am I tinkering with the gear?"* (see doodle). If we notice that we are tinkering with the safety gear (for example, checking and re-checking it to see how safe it is, making sure it's perfectly in order) then this might be a good sign that a bomb squad member is in town. There is likely to be some fear or discomfort up ahead. Something we are avoiding, and perhaps we are not even aware (yet) what that fear is. Our focus has become orientated towards safety, threat, protection. Our **PERFECTIONIST** is in charge, making sure everything is in order – ropes, harnesses, safety nets – and we are no longer enjoying the climb. Nor are we looking forward to the nice view that we might get when we reach the top.

ROCK CLIMBING METAPHOR

AM I TINKERING WITH
THE SAFETY GEAR
OR AM I
ENTOYING THE
VIEW ?

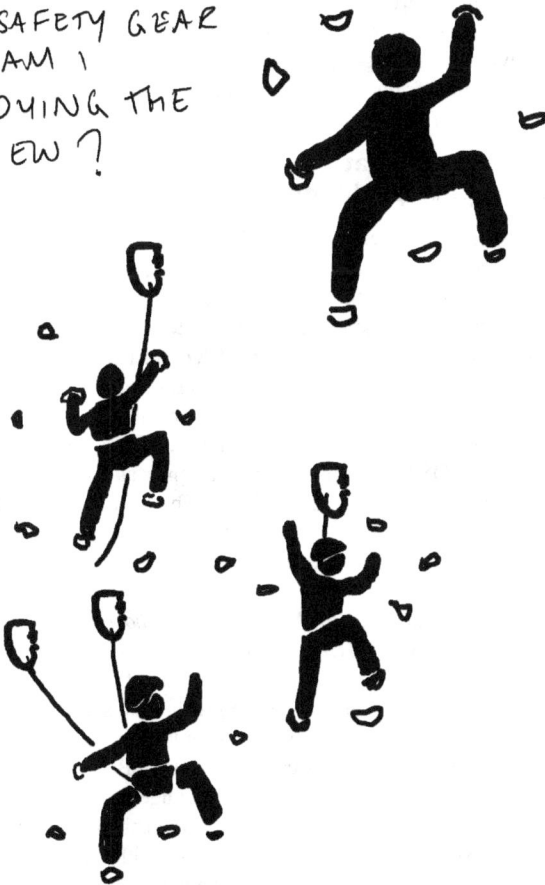

DOODLE: "Rock climbing metaphor"

In my writing, an example of me tinkering with the gear would be adjusting my fonts and margins back and forth and reading over every single sentence I have just written, to check each tiny part, one-by-one, before I can move on to the next. This is something I've caught myself doing hundreds of thousands of times. Perhaps more so earlier on in my career than I do now. Interestingly, it seems to be a lot more frequent when I'm doing academic writing than the kind of writing here in this book, where it feels more like I am talking to you, the reader. (I wonder if it's partly because, in this book, my main motivation is trying to help you, rather than to impress you!) In my work at Balanced Minds, there is an in-joke between me and my co-director, Chris (Irons), that whereas he can just trundle through answering his emails without too much fuss, I can take hours excruciating over each email until it is perfect. I am tinkering with my safety gear.

What are some of your examples of this in your own life?

PESSIMIST: to create low expectations and anticipate problems

The **PESSIMIST** is driven by similar fears to the **PERFECTIONIST** – they both fear failure. The types of explosions they use to avert this fear, however, are entirely different – almost the opposite in fact. While the **PERFECTIONIST** strives for meticulous standards and relentless attention to detail to make sure that errors and failure do not occur, the **PESSIMIST** either sets the bar so low that it's almost impossible to fail or even talks us out of starting the task in the first place. *"If you don't try at anything, you can't fail"* is one of its mantras. Not starting is the most assured and certain way to avoid failure, and so in the lead up before a task, the **PESSIMIST** will typically try to magnify all the things that could go wrong, and all the reasons why this task would be a waste of time. Drawing our attention to the worst has other protective functions too, even if we were to start the task. It keeps expectations low, not just our own self-expectations but also the expectations of others. *"It's nothing." "It's going to be rubbish." "Look at all these things that could go wrong." "Don't get your hopes up."*

Sometimes the **PESSIMIST** tries to create more of a safety net for us. So, it's not necessarily setting out to sabotage and halt our progress towards goals but more a precautionary measure *just in case* something goes wrong. There is good logic to this. If we set out with low expectations and then fail, then nothing's lost – we have matched expectation. But if we set out with low expectations and then succeed, if feels like a hugely rewarding (unexpected) win. Whereas setting out from an optimist position, there is a lot more at stake. With a high expectation, the two outcomes are either (i) a not particularly rewarding win (as it was expected), or (ii) a hugely distressing (unexpected) loss. In short, if a pessimist makes an error, it's a positive experience, whereas if an optimist makes an error, it's a negative experience.

It's partly because of this 'logic', that the **PESSIMIST** likes to think of itself as quite a realist, and quite a sensible advisor for us. But in truth, it is just playing things safe. And as we discovered with the **CERTAINTY-SEEKER**, playing it safe and staying within one's comfort zone can itself come with a cost, such as restricting our ability to grow, learn, and flourish. And what's more, the self-fulfilling prophecy can kick in to elicit self-defeating behaviour.

Our orientation towards pessimistic predictions of *"it's going to be rubbish"* and *"look at all these things that could go wrong"* will clearly start to influence our attention, our perceptions, our actions, which can ultimately shape the outcomes. So, what was perhaps intended as a safety net, can itself become the predominant driver and shaper of the outcomes.

As an example of how our **PESSIMIST** can result in self-sabotaging, let's consider the case of trying to quit smoking. So, my goal is quitting smoking, and my **PESSIMIST**, who is afraid that I might fail at this goal, will start throwing in a few safety nets for me, just in case I did fail to reach this goal. For example, it might start off by saying *"No chance". "Once a smoker, always a smoker"*. That way, if I failed at quitting, then at least I'd be ready and prepared with an explanation for why that happened, and it would be less likely to feel like a *personal* failure. (*"It's the addiction, not me"*). So, when I fail, I might feel disappointed, but at least I will have averted some of the more difficult (self-conscious) emotions like shame and embarrassment. The **PESSIMIST** might also remind me of all the times I've tried to quit in the past, which didn't work out. This, it thinks, will give me a bit of a cushion or soft landing when it doesn't work out this time either. *"You see, we've been here before." "Another year, same old story."*

We can already see how our safety net is starting to paint a picture for us, and is starting to shape the direction of travel. What we have essentially done here, in our attempts to avoid the fear of failure, is actually started laying ourselves a path towards failure!

Central to the **PESSIMIST**'s efforts is the motivation to protect us from the difficult feelings associated with failure, such as shame and embarrassment. And sometimes these efforts to avoid self-conscious emotions will lead it to magnifying and constructing external (non-self) causes of failure. It therefore overly focuses attention to problems, obstacles, and all the worst things that could happen. Once the 'failure' prediction is online, and is shaping perceptions, not only will we *perceive* more things as barriers (that we wouldn't have otherwise seen as barriers), but we might actively create new barriers to confirm the predictive model. In the smoking example, the predicted failure was attributed to 'my addiction', rather than to any personal failing of myself. So here, I created a story that allowed me to fail 'safely'.

This self-sabotaging controlled explosion is summarised below. Here we can see that the **PESSIMIST** is working so hard to protect us from our own feelings of failure that it inadvertently creates the optimum conditions for failure to happen.

HARM CREATED: *I create a 'failure' story that inadvertently lays a path to failure*

HARM AVERTED: *Fear of failure and experiencing shame and embarrassment*

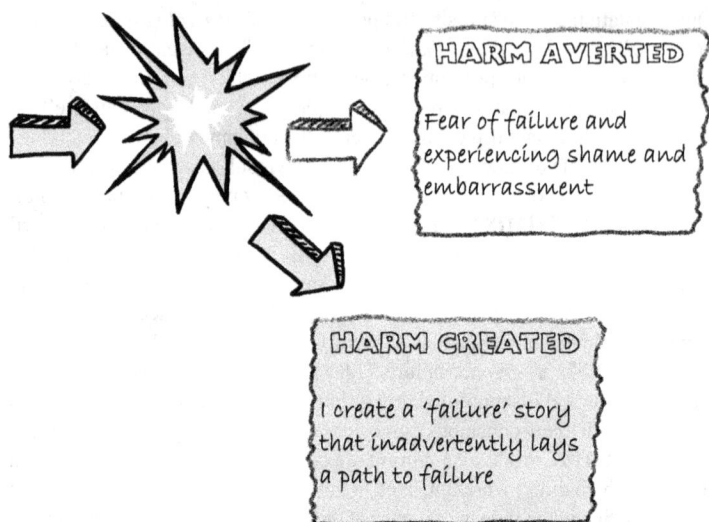

HARM AVERTED

Fear of failure and experiencing shame and embarrassment

HARM CREATED

I create a 'failure' story that inadvertently lays a path to failure

Pessimism to avoid failure-related shame and embarrassment

There may be times where our pessimistic predictions create self-sabotaging that goes even further than creating a perception and story about failure. For example, there might be times where we are actively constructing situations in which failure becomes more likely. With the smoking example, for instance, rather than waiting around for the predicted *'inevitable relapse'*, it might be that the person accelerates this process by starting an argument with their partner. The argument gets heated, both parties become stressed and angry, and then the person storms off out of the house to buy some cigarettes. Here, there are some direct actions that have fast-tracked and facilitated the failure story (*"We're going through a really stressful time in our relationship, so maybe now's not a good time to quit smoking after all"*).

Finally, to just think about some other areas of life in which this might play out: In relationships and dating, for example, if your **PESSIMIST** is saying *"This will end badly"*, do you think your interactions with this person will make it more or less likely to end badly? Although the **PESSIMIST** might be trying to give you a safety net (to lessen the pain in case you are rejected), it will also be actively shaping your perceptions and actions. As with all the other *controlled explosions* in this book (whether self-sabotaging, -criticising, or -harming), it is helpful for us to identify the trade-off – the trade-off between the harm created and the harm averted. And this gives us choices. *"What is more helpful here for me?" "Do I want to keep hold of my pessimism as a safety net?" "Or am I prepared to take a risk with some optimism?"*

There is no right or wrong answer to these questions. The empowerment here comes from an understanding of the trade-off and from the knowledge that we can choose.

CHAOS-CREATOR: to create drama, chaos, and catastrophe

In the Self-Sabotage Unit, we have so far met four members. Three of them use *controlled explosions* to keep things quite tight and ordered for us: the **CERTAINTY-SEEKER** wants us to exist in nice, predictable templates to help us navigate around the world; the **PERFECTIONIST** wants to make sure we are hyper-diligent with checking for errors; and the **PESSIMIST** wants to keep us in our comfort zone, where we're not at risk of failure. These three run quite a tight ship, they are quite controlling. The **PROCRASTINA-TOR**, unlike the other three, uses *controlled explosions* more as diversionary or distraction tactics – little tricks and hits of dopamine to woo us away from things we find difficult. The final unit member, the **CHAOS-CREATOR**, has a sprinkling of all these qualities: sometimes it uses *controlled explosions* to divert or distract attention away from something; at other times it may (counterintuitively) help to establish some order and control; and at other times it may even create a kind of hyper-alertness to, and action for, a particular issue that needs resolving.

Creating chaos to distract

Sometimes this happens in mid-life, maybe in your forties or fifties, when things are just starting to settle down – maybe you're in a settled home, you're married, your kids are at school, and you think, *"Oh. So, this is it? This is what I've been striving for and building up to for the last two or three decades? Right".* Maybe it's a sudden realisation that you are now middle-aged. Maybe you've been striving so hard for all those years that you have no idea of how to do 'settling down'. Maybe now that the dust has settled on all those years of building and striving, you're not sure if you have a purpose in life. Some deep questions start entering your mind. *"Am I in the right job?" "Have I made the right decisions?" "Is my marriage working?"* If we are feeling quite overwhelmed by these thoughts and feelings, our **CHAOS-CREATOR** might come along to the rescue: *"You don't want to be thinking about all that stuff. Let's shake things up a bit: Shall we move house? Move abroad? Have an affair? Get a new job?"*

In this scenario, the controlled explosion of chaos-creation is being used as a disrupter. It's a way of helping us avoid difficult feelings, questions, realisations, regrets, decisions. In that sense, we can think of it a bit like an extreme version of procrastination – a **PROCRASTINATOR** on steroids. It's not just a little distraction like checking social media for an hour or so, it's a truly explosive distraction that could grab and demand our attention for months, maybe years, to come.

There are of course more day-to-day versions of this. For example, sometimes we might create a drama or dilemma to avoid having a difficult conversation at home or with a colleague at work. "*I've been thinking, we really need to change over to a whole new IT system*" or "*we definitely need to rebrand our company with a new name*". Sometimes in politics, the government releases one headline-grabbing story on the same day as another, in an attempt to bury bad news. "*Look over there at this crisis*" (don't look over here).

Creating chaos to rediscover order

There is no better way to introduce this next idea than with a quote from Star Wars:

> "*One must destroy in order to create.*"

Yes, chaos and destruction are indeed chaotic and destructive. But only for a time. And then what happens next? And then after that? Sometimes it is helpful to think of chaos-creation not as an endpoint, but as a means to an end. The first step in a process.

As somebody who has always enjoyed listening to electronic dance music, I have become accustomed to some of the typical components in a dance track, as well as the emotional stages that a keen listener is taken through. There is usually a fair amount of predictability in things like when the changes and drops will occur. For example, each bar has four beats, and usually a small change happens every 4–8 bars, and then it's typically every 8–16 bars that something big, like the main drop, happens. The 4/8/16/32 bar loops continue throughout the track, so predictability is established. But then, before the drop, there is a protracted build-up stage, where tension is gradually increasing, with rushing percussion and snares (getting more and more cluttered and chaotic), before the heavy drop comes in with a strong, crisp, steady beat and bassline. The pleasurable and predictable release of the drop (i.e. the bit that makes you want to dance!) emerges out of the chaotic tension of the build-up.

The reason I mention this (apart from encouraging you to search up some 1990s UK drum and bass!) is to highlight that the chaotic tension is a necessary precursor to the pleasurable release. Without tension, there is no release. Without chaos-creation, there is no return to order. Earlier in this chapter, when we were exploring the edge (or sweet spot) between certainty and uncertainty (page 35), we considered the possible reasons why people may be attracted to venturing outside of their comfort zone.

One suggestion was that it may be rewarding to experience the resolution of, or developing mastery over, something uncertain. The same would equally apply to something chaotic. This leads us to consider, therefore, whether chaos-creation produces an opportunity for (rewarding) chaos-resolution. And if so, could it be that one of the functions of our inner **CHAOS-CREATOR** is to set up an experience of mastery?

It was also suggested that stepping outside our comfort zone – into the unknown – is necessary for learning and growth, linked to an innate human need to seek out novelty. It would have been essential for the survival of our evolutionary ancestors to courageously go out and explore. (Ancient people are known to have travelled a lot, discovering new climates, pastures, and locations to settle, and well as new fruits and animals to eat.) It could be that these two things are linked: the need to seek out novelty for growth and the need to develop mastery over uncertainty and chaos. So, returning to the *Star Wars* quote, *"one must destroy in order to create"*, could it be that our **CHAOS-CREATOR** is the catalyst for a growth process?

One of the main topics of Chapter 6 will be describing how *controlled explosions* can potentially be used for purposes of transformation and growth, but for this to happen, there needs to be an altogether different underlying motive to the one we are tracking in these earlier Chapters (1–5). In Paul Gilbert's three systems model [29], he describes our three basic survival life tasks and needs as: (i) harm avoidance, (ii) seeking out resources necessary for survival and reproduction, and (iii) rest and digest. We have so far been describing the bomb squad as being on a mission to protect – they create explosions to avert a feared harm from occurring. This is linked to the harm avoidance motivation. So when this basic motivational system is running the show, there is unlikely to be a broader vision of growth potential. Harm averted. Job done. As we saw in Chapter 1, our brain has evolved modules and algorithms to do certain jobs for us, and the job of the threat system is protection. So when this system is online, it creates a distinct psycho-physiological pattern that organises how we pay attention, think, feel, perceive, and behave. So, our perceptual and cognitive landscape becomes organised and shaped around the principle of 'better safe than sorry'. Within this limited landscape, it will be difficult to even *see* growth potential, let along pursue and action growth.

However, developing mastery over chaos could have benefits in more than one different motivational domain. On the threat-protection (harm avoidance) side, it could help us to get better at dealing with threats. And on the seeking/ pursuing side, it could help us to gain the courage and confidence to go out and explore. So the potential is definitely there for chaos to be a catalyst for building and growth, but the problem is the motivation. If we are primarily motivated and geared towards harm avoidance, then we might simply not be able see it. And this is where destructive patterns can be really harmful for us. With the threat system online, we can get caught in a spiral of self-destruction, and this can lead to all sorts of mental health problems, many of which will be covered in the following two chapters.

Creating chaos to enhance alertness and action for an issue that needs resolving

In the recent article I mentioned earlier, my colleague Tobyn and I present a *Perceptual Processing* account of voice-hearing, which describes situations of protective urgency whereby our brain might create a perception that "*amplifies* threat signals, *intensifies* emotions, and *escalates* responses" [11]. Here, an exaggerated, dramatised reality is created to elicit an action *to deal with* a particular threat. This contrasts with the scenario described previously, where something was created *to distract from* a threat. In this section we will explore how the **CHAOS-CREATOR** can sometimes serve as a stimulus for action. There is some cross-over here with the role of the **CATALYST**, who is a member of the Self-Harm Unit, because chaos, drama, and catastrophe can be a way to catalyse an urgency of response.

So how do we feel and experience chaos? Chaos produces a mixture of emotions for us, including anxiety, excitement, and suspense. There is an adrenaline rush. Our senses become alert and enhanced. We feel more 'alive'. It's invigorating. As already described, chaos creates a build-up of pressure and tension, and with that, grows a need and urge to reestablish order. Chaos demands quick thinking, and it demands some kind of action. These emotional and physical states could be appealing for someone, and in some circumstances, essential – especially if a person has found themselves quite trapped in a situation, or in a rut. Imagine, for example, someone who is stuck in indecision about their career. They're not enjoying their job, but at the same time they are scared about leaving it because, well, they need to pay the bills. This indecision is making them feel flat and depressed. They are growing exhausted from the ruminating about what they should or shouldn't do. This could be the type of situation where the bomb squad send in a **CHAOS-CREATOR**. The anticipated harm here is the fear of becoming trapped and depressed (maybe forever), and so the controlled explosion needs to create something that gives this person the spark, energy, and impetus to get themselves out of this rut. Maybe making a mistake at work? Maybe falling out with their boss? Something to clarify their decision making and catalyse their leaving. Hence, in this case, the controlled explosion is not a distraction, it is a catalyst for protective action.

HARM CREATED: *I create a problem or fall-out at work that speeds up my decision to leave*

HARM AVERTED: *Crippling indecision about my job and fear of being trapped/depressed*

It may sound counterintuitive, the notion of chaos providing clarity! How can a state of chaos provide resolution to a problem? It depends entirely on how you define the problem. Here the problem is not the actual career decision per se, it is the state of *stuckness*. The chaos has not provided a correct answer to the question "what is the right or wrong career choice for me?". Who knows? Maybe there is no answer to that question. Like most things in life, there is no clear right or wrong. But what the controlled explosion has provided is a solution to the problem of *stuckness* – the harmful and debilitating experience of indecision and impasse. It was a psychological-emotional state that needed resolving.

In this example, a controlled explosion was created in the external world (i.e. in their job-related relationships and actions) to initiate the direction forward. There may also be an equivalent process that happens in our internal world – psychologically: a controlled explosion that creates a kind of internal chaos in our own mind. One area of my own academic research has been focused on people who report having 'anomalous experiences'. (*Anomalous* means unusual or somehow deviating from the normal. I've sometimes preferred the term, '*out-of-the-ordinary*'.) These experiences, which occur throughout the population [12, 30] are sometimes attributed to spiritual, mystical, or psychic phenomena. At other times, they are attributed to being signs of a psychiatric condition such as psychosis.

In one of our earliest studies, we interviewed people from both clinical and non-clinical populations about the nature and onset of their out-of-the-ordinary experiences [31]. Our research team found that in most of our small sample of 12 (6 clinical, 6 non-clinical), these experiences had first emerged at a point in their life where they had been experiencing *emotional suffering* (11 of 12 people) and *existential questioning* (8 of 12 people). The existential questioning typically involved "deep personal thinking and questioning about the meaning and/or direction of life", often prompted by a feeling that they had reached an impasse or dead-end in their lives.

These research findings add support to the idea that, in the right circumstances, our brain might create a controlled explosion to help us get out of an emotional rut. This could take the form of an anomalous perceptual experience – the psychological equivalent of a 'chaos', in that it has very similar qualities to the experience of chaos described above: novelty, disorientation, fear, absorption, excitement, adrenaline, heightened senses, and so on.[1] In these cases, we can think of this as our internal **CHAOS-CREATOR** shaking things up for us (psychologically, existentially) to help us move forward from a stuck place. Other researchers in this same field have described this process as a kind of existential problem-solving [32].

HARM CREATED: *Anomalous experience*

HARM AVERTED: *At a dead-end (impasse) in life, with no sense of purpose or direction*

Creating chaos to feel alive: sensation-seeking

I briefly mentioned sensation-seeking earlier in this chapter, when we were focusing on the 'tug-of-war' we can often find ourselves in between familiarity and novelty; between the known and the unknown; between certainty-seeking and sensation-seeking. The **CHAOS-CREATOR** is most certainly someone you'd want on your tug-of-war team if you were on the sensation-seeking side. Chaos will bring sensations galore! Up to this point, we have been considering examples of where chaos-creation can be a means to an end (i.e. to distract, to rediscover order, or to resolve problems that are stuck). However, when we consider its sensation-heightening qualities, we can also appreciate that sometimes chaos-creation can be an end in itself for people. Sensation-seeking can make us feel alive. It can become addictive. The **CHAOS-CREATOR** can simply become a way of living and being, not specifically linked to avoiding harm. It could of course be linked to an avoidance at some level, for example, avoiding monotony and boredom. But not necessarily. It could be linked to a philosophy, a value, or belief. Hedonism, for example, is a philosophy that life should be about maximising pleasure. So there may be people who see every day as a new opportunity to feel more sensations. Creating chaos and unpredictability could be sought after as a way of life.

> *"We imagine war is tough. We know it puts great strain on soldiers. But is war a drug?"*
>
> (Quote from the film, The Hurt Locker)

In this quoted film, *The Hurt Locker*, we see how soldiers can become addicted to the adrenaline rush of being in extremely dangerous and unpredictable situations. (This film also happens to be about a bomb squad in a war zone, although that's an aside, and not the reason for mentioning it here.) There are other more day-to-day versions of seeking sensation through chaos. Think about art. Many artists aim to create paradoxical perceptions through their artwork. They can successfully elicit visual chaos and contradiction in the minds of their audience, which can evoke interest and fascination. It's intriguing. Think also about spicy food, which can create chaos in our mouths and taste buds. Over time, we can learn to love (and crave more of) that burning sensation in our mouths. With music, too, we might long for some discordant sounds that hook us in through their auditory chaos. We are gripped by TV drama series that end their episodes on a 'cliff-hanger'. We listen to 'edgy' podcasters and comedians who leave us feeling shocked and perplexed: *'I cannot believe they just said that. Wow, that is actually what they said'* (accompanied by slight thrill and excitement to have heard this extreme utterance that's broken all social rules and norms). Those are some of the day-to-day versions of controlled chaos that create sensations for us. Can you think of any others that spice things up in your life?

Guilty pleasures

The idea of guilty pleasures is interesting, because there seems to be a dual motivation here. Am I seeking a feeling of pleasure and satisfaction? Or am I seeking the thrill of uncertainty as to whether or not I will be punished for doing something wrong? These are both 'good feelings', but one is more linked to contentment and the other more to excitement. Even better if it's both together! If I eat that whole tub of ice cream while lying in bed, I will have both the feeling of being naughty, rebellious (flirting with some kind of social danger, perhaps) whilst also having the inner warmth and contentment (as my body welcomes the smooth creamy textures and pleasurable flavours).

The rewarding nature of the pleasure part of a 'guilty pleasure' might be more obvious. The guilty part is a bit more complex and requires a bit more attention for this book on controlled explosions. *Guilty* implies that I have done something wrong or bad. Some sense that I will be judged by others for this action, some negative social evaluation (if they found out). There may be some social guilt or shame involved. There may also be a link here to what we were saying before about listening to 'edgy' podcasters or comedians. The shock of the edginess, and the thrill of engaging with material that steps outside the boundaries of what is socially acceptable. So, at some level, this might also be driven by a desire to challenge the authority. A rebellion. A bit like how a child pushes the boundary of their parent or teacher. Hence, there might be some expression of anger at the heart of this – a way of protesting against parents or society more generally. *"I'm going to eat this whole tub of ice cream, and there's not a damn thing you can do about it."* We will spend more time in Chapters 3 and 4 considering situations in which anger (or suppressed anger) may contribute to controlled explosions. Some people may of course seek their sensations through crime, rioting, and creating public disorder. Disruptive behaviour can be a version of chaos-creation, where the excitement and thrill come through the uncertainty of *"Am I going to get into trouble?"* (for example, with the Police or some other authority figure).

This is interesting when thinking about addictions. We often talk about the substances themselves (such as street drugs) as being addictive, and our society often thinks that the best way to help people with addictions is to ban these substances and make them harder to get hold of by making them illegal. We also create legal punishments for people, so that they know they're doing something bad or wrong. But what if the addictive lure of the drug was not so much the effect of the drug, but the process of using the drug? The more illegal and wrong it is, the more uncertainty, thrill, adrenaline I feel. Maybe I'll be caught and punished. Maybe not. How far can I go with this? How close can I sail to the wind here? I'm addicted to the thrill of how far I can take my drug use and the uncertainty of whether I will be punished. For many, particularly in the early days, drug use can serve all these functions, from thrill and sensation-seeking, to challenging authority, to a form of guilty pleasure.

In Appendix 3, there are some worksheets you can use for mapping out your own examples of self-sabotaging controlled explosions. There is also step-by-step guidance (with examples) to help you with the choices you can make once you have identified these in your life.

Note

1 If you are interested in learning more about the types of anomalous experiences that people report, Appendix 2 lists the full 19 items of a scale that we developed for detecting these in the general population: the *Transpersonal Experiences Questionnaire* (TEQ).

Chapter 3

Self-Criticism Unit

Controlled explosions that can harm us psychologically

Chapter summary

This chapter explores forms and functions of self-criticism. Some versions of self-criticism are more focused on our flaws and inadequacies, while others are more self-disliking and self-hating. Some people have extremely hostile internal abusers, which may or may not remind them of memories and relationships with real people from their past lives. Some members of our Self-Criticism Unit want us to improve and do better, and others seem to want to attack us or cause us harm. This chapter will consider some of the different types of self-criticism and some of the interesting models and ideas to help us understand why they occur. It will explore some possible functions of self-criticism and, again, consider what might be the 'bigger harms' that are being avoided or prevented.

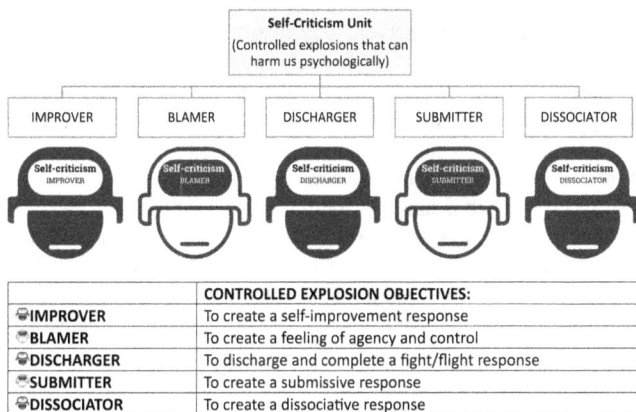

	Self-Criticism Unit (Controlled explosions that can harm us psychologically)			
IMPROVER	BLAMER	DISCHARGER	SUBMITTER	DISSOCIATOR
Self-criticism IMPROVER	Self-criticism BLAMER	Self-criticism DISCHARGER	Self-criticism SUBMITTER	Self-criticism DISSOCIATOR

	CONTROLLED EXPLOSION OBJECTIVES:
IMPROVER	To create a self-improvement response
BLAMER	To create a feeling of agency and control
DISCHARGER	To discharge and complete a fight/flight response
SUBMITTER	To create a submissive response
DISSOCIATOR	To create a dissociative response

Members, roles, and objectives of the Self-Criticism Unit

DOI: 10.4324/9781003559924-6

We usually think of a relationship as something we have with other people, not with ourselves. But actually the relationship we have with ourselves is one of the most important we will ever have. It's the only relationship that we will be living with every second of every day for our whole life. What kind of relationship do you have with yourself? Maybe it changes from situation to situation. How do you relate to yourself when you are struggling? How do you relate to yourself when you make a mistake? Sometimes we can be quite self-critical, especially when we mess up or when we are finding something difficult. For example, we might say to ourselves "get a grip" or "for goodness sake, sort it out". We might curse or swear at ourselves or call ourselves insulting names. In this chapter we will explore how this self-to-self relationship can sometimes become recruited for creating our *controlled explosions*, whereby one part of us becomes a harm-creator, and in turn, another part becomes the receiver of this harm. Essentially our brain is playing out both roles in a harmful relationship – it is switching on a relational pattern where one part of us starts to criticise, shame or even attack another part of ourselves. While this might not sound particularly pleasant, one thing I hope we have learnt by now about *controlled explosions* is that the harms created by our brains are often crucial and necessary (albeit unpleasant) to prevent an even greater feared or predicted harm.

Before we get into some of the roles and workings of the Self-Criticism Unit, let's first explore the mechanisms of why we even have a self-to-self relationship in the first place. According to evolutionary theory, we have brains that evolved to be useful for our survival. If you recall from Chapter 1, our evolved brains even shape our perceptual experience of the world in a way that is survival-enhancing, as opposed to perceiving the reality of what's there. Our brains are survival machines, and they have developed a range of functions and patterns that support this goal. That is their primary purpose, and indeed everything that our brain can do – from perceiving, to feeling, to thinking, to imagining, to dreaming – is only there because it's helped our species to survive in some way or other. Survival overrides everything. Even at the expense of seeing the world accurately. Even at the expense of feeling happy and content. And as we will see in this chapter, one of the big costs of having a survival-obsessed brain is that many of us have to live our lives with a resident inner bully – our self-critic.

One of the clever ways that our brain has helped us survive is by organising itself into patterns that support the formation of social relationships. We are a social species, which means that forming relationships (caring, attachment, connection, and working together) has been an important survival strategy for our ancestors. In a world full of danger, the ancestors who were better at forming groups or tribes would have had a far better chance of survival than the ancestors who left the group or ventured out alone into the wilderness. So having a brain that orientated us towards social relating was a good thing. To do this, what's required is being born with brains that are equipped with templates of what social relationships are like and how social roles work. When we are born, we need a built-in template of what a caring relationship is like and we also need a template of what a hostile relationship is like. Additionally, within each of these templates, we need to have a model or 'map' of each role within the relationship. So for a caring relationship, we need to have a prototype of both a care-giver and a care-receiver. For a hostile relationship, we need to have a prototype of both a harm-giver and a harm-receiver. These are all etched into our brains from before we are born. Remember, in an evolutionary sense, the ancestors who were quick to discern a hostile person or gesture from one that is caring would have been more likely to survive and pass on their genes. This means that they had to have more effective templates/prototypes of hostility versus caring from which to discern.

The term used by Paul Gilbert for these built-in templates is *social mentalities* [33]. Social mentalities organise our relationships, and each social mentality contains within it a representation of both roles within the relationship. To organise caring relationships, for example, the social mentality contains a profile of both the care-giver and care-receiver. In a power relationship, the social mentality contains a profile of both the powerful/dominant and the powerless/subordinate. However, a key insight from Gilbert's work [29, 33] is the recognition that social mentalities not only switch on to organise relationships with other people, but they can also pattern and texture the relationships we have with ourself. So, for example, we can switch on the caring mentality when we are being self-caring and self-compassionate (i.e. we are in the dual roles of both care-giver and care-receiver). We can also switch on threat-giving and threat-receiving mentalities, for example, when we are being critical, condemning, and harmful towards ourselves. In this moment, we are both the giver and receiver of threat – we are simultaneously sending hostile signals to ourselves, as well as responding in a protective way to this hostility.

So now that we have outlined the mechanisms behind our brains' ability to form self-to-self relationships, we can focus our attention more closely on these self-critical ways of relating and the relevance of self-criticism to *controlled explosions*. In the Self-Criticism Unit of the bomb squad, there are quite a range of differences in how they go about their work. Sometimes the self-criticism is about wanting us to improve and do better, while at other times it's more about wanting to harm, punish, or attack us. In the *Forms of Self-Criticising/Attacking & Self-Reassuring Scale* (FSCRS), Gilbert and colleagues distinguish between forms of self-criticism that focus on a sense of personal inadequacy and those that convey a desire to hurt or persecute the self [34].

In this chapter, I will differentiate between five types of self-critic which correspond not to the focus of the criticism, but to the feelings and responses elicited. As mentioned previously, there are two roles within the self-critical relationship – both the giver and receiver of the criticism. While most previous literature has focused on the criticism-giving role (it's focus, such as on inadequacies of self or hatred of self), in this book, I will shift the focus more to the criticism-receiving role (it's impact, such as on the feelings and actions elicited). As we will see, this shift of focus will help us later when it comes to understanding what might be going on in terms of *controlled explosions*.

These are five subtypes of self-critic within the bomb squad, each with a slightly different role in terms of the impact they are aiming to elicit in us:

- Improver – to create a self-improvement response
- Blamer – to create a feeling of agency and control
- Discharger – to discharge and complete a fight/flight response
- Submitter – to create a submissive response
- Dissociator – to create a dissociative response.

IMPROVER: to create a self-improvement response

The self-critic that demands to get an improvement out of us (the proverbial kick up the backside) is perhaps the version most familiar to many of us. On the surface, this critic is on our side, rooting for us, coaching us, and wanting us to reach our potential. Indeed, many of us are desperate to cling on to this critic and are terrified by the thought of not having it or letting it go. However, the more we dig into this, we can see that often the motivation is located (as with the other *controlled explosions*) in averting some feared harm from happening. Consider the example of a self-critic that says:

> *"Why do you keep messing this up? Come on, you've really got to sort yourself out. This is the fifth bloody time this has happened now. There was that time on Tuesday where you ..."* [and continues to relay the list of mistakes that have been logged]

So, on the one hand, this critic seems motivated to help. It wants to see an improvement, which is probably very much in line with what you want to see too. However, a key question is *why* it wants to see this improvement. Is it because it is motivated to give a boost to your well-being? Or is it motivated by the fear of what could happen if you weren't to improve? If you kept making these mistakes, what's the worst that could happen? What if your mistakes were seen by others as inadequacies? What if it became obvious to others that you are flawed in some way? What if they started to talk about or laugh about these flaws behind your back? What if they started to distance themselves from you? What if you ended up socially rejected and alone? The more that fears and threats are 'heating' the self-critic in the background, the more intense and insistent the self-critic will become. The self-critic might be incessantly trying to highlight your flaws to you before they are found out by others.

> **HARM CREATED:** *Pointing out my mistakes, flaws, inadequacies to myself*

> **HARM AVERTED:** *Other people seeing my mistakes, flaws, and inadequacies*

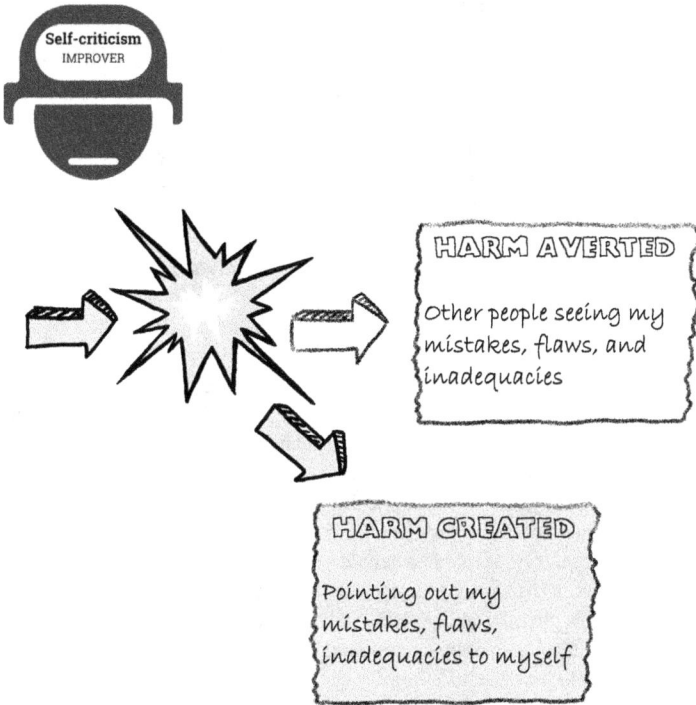

A self-critic aiming to elicit self-improvement by pointing out my flaws

The underlying fears will likely be fuelling the nature of the self-critic, for example, making its tone louder, shaping its emotional texture, making the self-critical words and messages more direct, blunt, and attention-grabbing. ("You're a fucking useless piece of shit", for example, is more likely to make you pay attention than "oh I really don't think that's a good way of going about it".) Just like the school playground bully, the fear-fuelled self-critic is likely to go for the most blunt and effective route of making an impact on you – giving you a jolt so that you wake up to the importance of this need to self-improve, before something terrible happens. Self-improve or else. In Compassion Focused Therapy, there is a helpful distinction often made between a *self-critic* and a *compassionate self-corrector*. It is of course important for all of us to self-improve, but the key is what is the motivational tone and texture behind this. When we have a self-critic as our self-improvement coach, it is more likely this is being driven by fear and harm-avoidance than by a desire for well-being, flourishing, and growth.

Another thing that greatly influences how this improvement-seeking critic goes about its work is our past experiences and relationships with other people – particularly our parents, teachers, and other authority figures who were involved with trying to improve us and making us grow into better humans. When it's our threat system that is driving our self-critic, then our brains will automatically link up all threat-based memories of being criticised in the past, and all the worst mistakes we've made that have displeased our superiors the most. Our self-to-self relationships are often a playing out of past relationships that have been attached to our (built-in) social mentalities. Sometimes the content of the self-critic is directly linked to words and tones that we have in our memory of these (earlier) interactions. Sometimes the content is not linked to personal memory, but perhaps linked to archetypal images, figures, tones, and to characters in fairytales, cartoons, books, and movies.

The theory of social mentalities is closely aligned to Carl Jung's work around the archetypes of the collective unconscious, which are inherited patterns in our minds shared by all of us. Therefore, the social mentality of a critical relationship (which, remember, encompasses both roles – the giver and receiver of the criticism) may contain clusters of images, themes, words that are not from personal life/memory but more the evolved/archetypal patterns. You may have noticed that when you dream there is often content in your dreams that you have never seen before. Our brain has a wonderful capacity for imagination, and can give us new content. This is great for authors like Stephen King who can make a very successful career tapping into the darkest corners of our collective imagination. But when it comes to the self-critic, these imaginary powers can really work against us and cause us a great amount of self-directed harm. This can be devastating for our mental health, but certainly can make for a highly effective controlled explosion.

It may be that the degree of controlled explosion will be related to the level of feared harm that would otherwise come by not improving. At one end of the continuum, if there is a mild fear, my critic might be saying "come on Charlie, you can do better than this", but as the degree of fear rises, the self-critic might increase in intensity, volume, persistence. At higher levels of fear the self-critic might start swearing at me, and the *controlled explosions* they create may recruit images and sounds from my memories of being criticised in the past. At other times, my self-critic might create a controlled explosion from archetypal images of criticism and power, which I might even experience as being externally generated. We will return to this in Chapter 5 ('remote detonators'), but just to briefly mention here, in my therapy practice I have worked with many people who experience their criticism and attacks as coming from an external source – these people, who have often received a diagnosis of psychosis, are hearing critical voices being spoken to or about them. They may also be seeing demonic visions in front of them and may be sensing the presence of hostile others. In Chapter 5, I will explore the possibility that perhaps these remotely detonated controlled explosions are an *even more* effective way of grabbing our attention, and perhaps that these kinds of controlled explosion are used for averting the most extreme fears of harm.

BLAMER: to create a feeling of agency and control

This member of the bomb squad is tasked with the job of attributing blame to us, particularly for everything bad that happens. *"It's your fault." "The reason that this has happened is down to your own uselessness or mistakes." "This problem is of your own making."* If this self-critic is left to carry on in this way over time, this could lead to more entrenched feelings of shame *("I'm a bad person"*, or someone *"flawed"* or *"defective"*). So what is this type of self-critic up to? Could there be a protective function of attributing blame to ourselves? Let's consider a few scenarios where a self-blaming approach might be the least bad option.

Self-blame can create a feeling of agency and control

In some situations, it may be adaptive to believe that it's your fault, even when it isn't. Take the example of a young child who is desperately seeking the love and attention of their parent, but their parent is far too busy with work to notice the child's need. There are two options for child to make sense of this situation: the first option is to blame the parent, and the second option is to blame themselves. In a child's eye, not only is the first option very hard to conceive (with their very limited understanding of the world, of work, and of the balance of competing responsibilities), but this option is also potentially very dangerous and scary for them. If it is the parent who is responsible, then the 'unmet needs' experience is entirely out of the child's control. They are utterly helpless and powerless to whether 'met needs' is something that happens, and of course there is the terrifying possibility of this never happening. The second option, however – this is my own fault – at least leaves a glimmer of hope that there may be something I can influence. If only I was a better kid, then I would be loved. If only I was less annoying, made fewer mistakes, or changed myself somehow, then I might become loveable to that parent. I might win that love over time. So, whereas the first option (parent-blame) rendered the child helpless, the second option (self-blame) provides an orientation and a path forward. With this comes a sense of agency, purpose, and control.

Self-blame can avert competitive emotions (like anger) and conflict

We will stay with the child example above and think a bit more about that first option (parent-blame). I highlighted previously the helplessness that the child might feel if they were to conceive the parent as being at fault. For a young child, in whose eyes the parent is almost God-like, the concept itself might not even arise. But at a certain age, a child might (rightly) attribute fault to the parent and might (rightly) feel anger towards that parent. There may be a sense that this is not fair, an angry emotional energy may be igniting in their body, and with an urge to protest. This is where the child is faced with another two difficult options. The first option is to express and direct their anger towards the parent. The second option is to redirect the angry emotional energy somewhere else. The first option here is very risky for a child. They rely on their parent, and need them for, well ..., everything. Can they really risk a confrontation or conflict? What if the parent retaliated, either an angry response of their own, or by proceeding to deny or withhold more love from their child – for example, by closing the door and becoming more engrossed in this thing they call "work". For the child, it may be too risky to go any further down that path of parent-blame, anger, conflict, and the fear that this might make things worse. And yet there is still this angry emotion alive in the child's body. It is building like a pressure-cooker and has no outlet and nowhere to go. How does the child discharge this energy? It may be possible to suppress or numb this emotion, for example, by pushing it down into their body so that it is no longer part of their conscious awareness. Or another possibility is to redirect it towards a different target – the self.

Self-blaming critic to the rescue! The danger has been averted, however, in this case, the self-critic is also fuelled with a brimming tank of angry energy needing to be released. The self-directed blame might therefore come with a certain amount of 'flavour' to it – a hostile tone, an insulting intent, some angry words and phrases that the child might have heard before. In the same way that the self-improvement critic might intensify according to the level of fear, the self-blaming critic might intensify according to the level of anger.

The self is not the only target available for anger that needs redirecting. For some children, it can be other children or siblings, often younger siblings, who come into the firing line. Essentially the angry emotion is looking for a home. It is not safe to be housed in the child–parent relationship, where the parent has all the power. It may be safer housed in the self-to-self relationship or in a relationship with someone less powerful.

DISCHARGER: to discharge and complete a fight/flight response

Some critic-initiated controlled explosions may be targeting the past. This is like the Second World War bomb in Bermondsey that hasn't detonated. There are a load of potential chemical reactions that are frozen in time – from inside an old Second World War bomb to inside the body after trauma. In school days, I remember from my physics lessons that a basic rule of energy is that it cannot be created or destroyed, it can only be converted from one form to another. This is called 'the law of conservation of energy' and means that the energy contained in a closed system always remains constant. There are however, two main forms of energy: kinetic and potential. Kinetic energy is energy in motion, whereas potential energy is energy that is stored in an object, ready to produce kinetic energy later on. Food has potential energy, measured by calories (kcal), which is stored inside the food ready to be converted into kinetic energy for our body to operate. The potential (chemical) energy is stored in the food's sugars, and when the food is broken down, it becomes transferred or metabolised into kinetic energy (thermal and mechanical energy, for heat and movement). Another example of potential energy is an archer's longbow. Think about the potential energy that is stored in the stretched elastic string as the archer takes aim. And then the conversion of potential to kinetic energy that occurs upon releasing the arrow. Okay, that's enough of the physics lesson!

There are times when we, as humans, might activate an energy sequence, but cannot complete the cycle. So, to break this down, here are the steps:

1   We perceive a threat in the environment
2   Our body initiates the threat response by releasing cortisol (a hormone that regulates the body's metabolism and energy) to prepare energy for fight-or-flight
3   It is too dangerous to convert this energy into muscle movements and actions, and so we must keep it stored in the body.

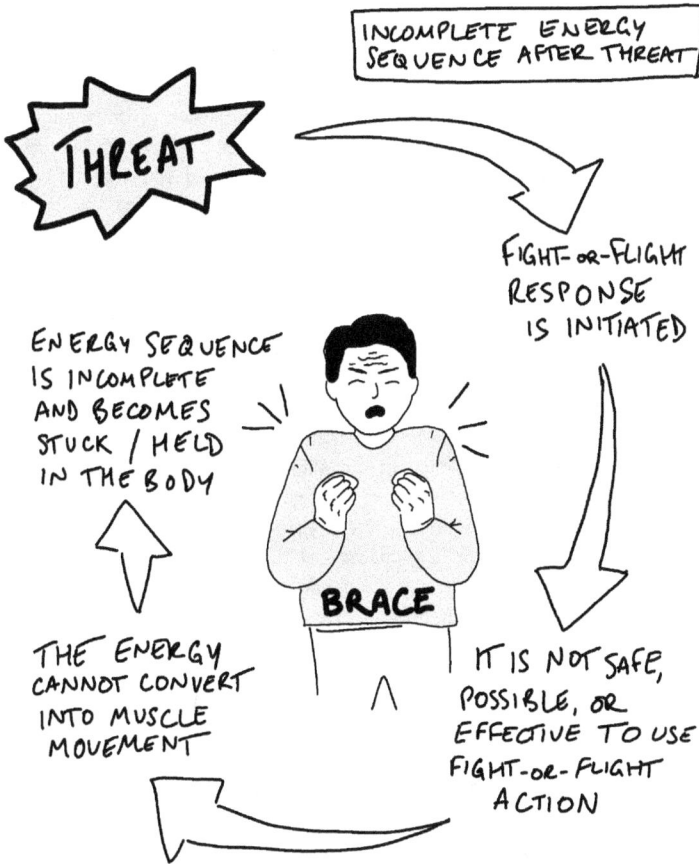

DOODLE: "Incomplete energy sequence after threat"

There are several prominent trauma theories that centre around the idea of uncompleted fight-or-flight responses that are held in the body. For example, both Somatic Experiencing therapy (Peter Levine) and Sensorimotor Psychotherapy (Pat Ogden) aim to treat people with trauma and PTSD by helping them to discharge and complete their bodies' (pent-up) threat responses that were obstructed at the time of trauma. Imagine that our archer was frozen in that moment just before releasing the arrow. A movement sequence has already been initiated. Chemical energy (food) has already been converted into thermal and mechanical energy for external work (body and muscle movement). The energy is on the cusp of being transferred into the arrow as an external discharge, but the cycle has not been completed. Where does that energy now go? Some of the energy can be released as heat (thermal energy), but there are still large amounts of movement (mechanical energy) that have to be either rerouted somewhere else in the body or stored somewhere in the body to be released and discharged later on.

With threat situations, there is an even higher state of arousal – my body is stuck in a state of readiness for either fight (anger) or flight (escape). Perhaps, if I could just get through to the end of today, then some of this trapped energy could be released later when I am asleep and dreaming. If I am lucky, my brain might be able to construct me a dream in which the same emotion can be aroused (anger or fear), the response can be mobilised, and the energy released. Ok, I might wake up in the morning sweating after a turbulent night of dreams, but at least the cycle is now completed. The emotion is processed, and my nervous system can now settle.

The body-based trauma theories regard PTSD symptoms (such as flashbacks) as the body's attempts to 'complete' the cycle. The trauma memory is being re-experienced as sensory intrusions, flashbacks, and nightmares. The same understanding could be applied to some types of self-critic, particularly those which resemble what Kate Lucre calls "abuser echoes" [28]. In the bomb squad, the **DISCHARGER** critic may be using *controlled explosions* to arouse an (incomplete) threat response that needs to be processed.

Here, again, we have a paradox of something in our brain that is both helpful and harmful (simultaneously). There is a self-generated explosion that obviously causes us a great deal of psychological harm – it may be activating strong emotions like hatred, anger, and disgust, and channelling these emotions and harmful intent towards us. It is not hard to see why many people would conclude that this critic is not welcome and *does not belong* in me. Something we might want to push away and get rid of. However, what if we held in mind that our brain might be attempting to complete a trauma memory? In the same way that our brain might give us an anxious or angry dream to help us process a life event. What if we also held in mind the costs (possibly even greater harms) of not completing the emotion – of continuing to exist in a body that is holding uncompleted threat. Some of this harm could be physical, such as body tension, pain, and even illness or disease.

HARM CREATED: *Attacks to switch on threat emotions and responses (fight/flight)*

HARM AVERTED: *Pent-up emotions and undischarged responses that may cause disease*

In Gabor Maté's popular book, *When the Body Says No: The Cost of Hidden Stress*, he presents a scientific argument for the contribution of suppressed emotions (in particular, anger) to a range of chronic physical illnesses and diseases, such as arthritis, heart disease, and cancer.

> *The anxiety of anger and other 'negative' emotions like sadness and rejection may become deeply bound in the body. Eventually it is transmitted into biological changes through the multiple and infinitely subtle cross-connections of the PNI apparatus, the unifying nexus of body/mind. This is the route that leads to organic disease. When anger is disarmed, so is the immune system. Or when the aggressive energy of anger is diverted inward, the immune system becomes confused. Our physiological defences no longer protect us or may even turn mutinous, attacking the body.*

(Gabor Maté [35])

SUBMITTER: to create a submissive response

This bomb squad member plays an important protective role – it is a creator of our submissive response. It jumps into action when the safest thing for us to do is to yield, surrender, or become compliant to a superior force. This is particularly useful when we cannot fight or escape from a person who has power over us, or in other situations where we have to accept our powerless position. This self-critic achieves a submissive response in us by playing out the powerful–powerless relationship in our own brains. It takes the role of a powerful authority, often using loud and aggressive language, tones, or even threats to assert its power. In that moment, our brain is playing out both sides of a power relationship. One part of us is the 'dominant' giver of criticism, and another part is the 'subordinate' receiver of this. In other words, our brain has a clever way of stimulating itself into submissiveness.

Self-submission to avoid harm, humiliation, and trauma

In what situations would it be helpful to have an internal (built-in) submission-maker? Well, of course, as with all bomb squad missions, it comes down to averting an even bigger anticipated harm. If I can submit (myself) before I even encounter a harm, then I won't have to go through the painful, perhaps humiliating, experience of having to submit to a person who is more powerful than me. If I am a trauma survivor who has experienced real harm from people in my life, my brain will be particularly attuned to protecting me from ever having to go through a similar traumatising experience again. When describing how trauma can affect our minds and lives, the author Daniela Sieff suggests that "we are not only frightened of being retraumatised, we are also frightened of losing control" and that "our lives become organised around the imperative to avoid anything that might trigger these emotions" [36]. So self-elicited submission can be a highly effective way of avoiding situations where we might experience harm, humiliation, and even trauma and re-traumatisation.

HARM CREATED: *Self criticise/attack which elicits inferior feelings and submissive responses*

HARM AVERTED: *The likelihood of being a target of harm from other people*

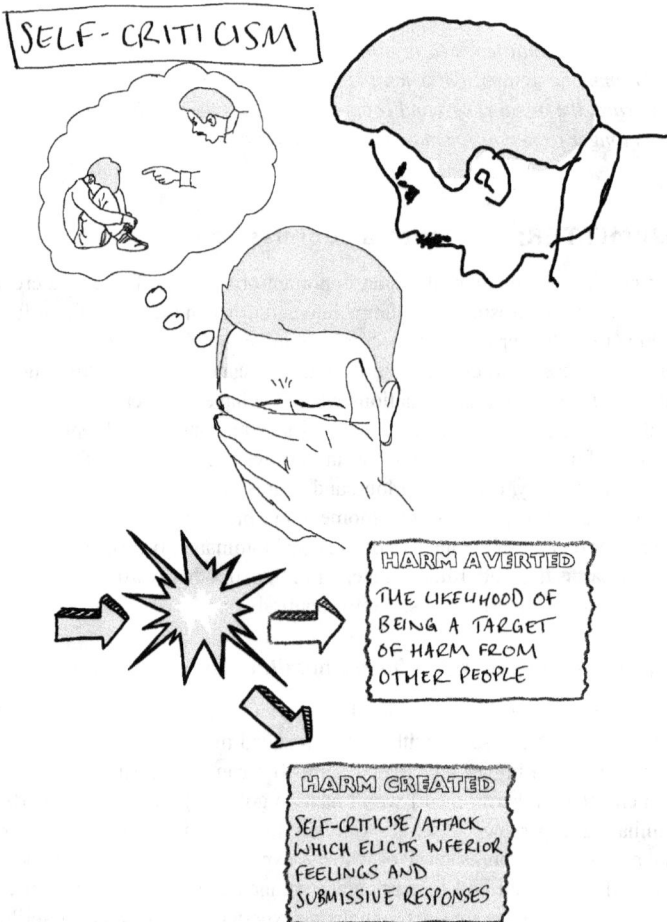

SELF-CRITICISM

HARM AVERTED
THE LIKELIHOOD OF BEING A TARGET OF HARM FROM OTHER PEOPLE

HARM CREATED
SELF-CRITICISE/ATTACK WHICH ELICITS INFERIOR FEELINGS AND SUBMISSIVE RESPONSES

DOODLE: "Self-criticism"

Self-submission to avoid competitive emotions like anger

Our internal submission-maker is also an effective bomb squad member for avoiding conflict and our own feelings of anger. Here there is overlap with some roles of the self-blaming critic introduced previously. Indeed, self-blame could be a route towards self-submission. I have met many people who are not comfortable with their own anger. Some people are experts at avoiding arguments and confrontation. Some people I have heard say, "I don't do anger", or for a couple, you might hear them say, "oh we never argue". I have even met people who wear this as a badge of honour, as if there is some pride of managing to conquer ever allowing their angry feelings to emerge.

I can certainly empathise with this myself – for many years of my life, I have fitted into a mould and identity as an easy-going, chilled-out person. For many years this had generally felt like a massive compliment and something that I aspired to. But I later came to realise that it was quite restrictive for me. If I am always the chilled-out guy, where is the room for my anger? What if people take advantage of my easy-going nature? What if everyone assumes, "oh I'm sure Charlie will be cool with that" and then maybe I'm not? If I have angry energy switching on in my body, this will feel very at odds with how I am seen by others, and how I am seen by myself. Can I risk letting this emotion be seen by others? Can I risk letting myself even feel this emotion? If I feel it, I might need to own it. And if I own it, I might need to act on it or do something. Tell you what, let's just not risk it. Let's just keep things as they are – easy-going. However, to do this, I'm going to need to call on my internal bomb squad. In fact, there are a few roles here that my bomb squad members can help with:

A Help me avoid situations where there might be a chance I could feel angry
B If I am in an unavoidable situation where I might feel angry, help me to avoid a conflict or confrontation with this person
C If I do feel angry, help me to redirect or channel this away from the other person.

My inner submission-making critic can help me with all three. To help me with (A), my self-critic can switch on and start attacking me with insults and threats before I have even left my home. The defeat–submission response is therefore activated in me long before I even get close to the situation. The most effective self-critics may even start up before we have got out of bed in the morning, keeping us under the duvet all day and well away from any potential conflict. Those of you readers who have experienced depression may be familiar with this – that feeling of waking up with a strong sense of defeat, with no interest to get up, nothing to look forward to, and no motivation to leave the home. The self-critic can indeed contribute to and maintain depression through this eliciting of defeat states (for a review of the research linking defeat and depression, see Taylor and colleagues [37]).

To help me with (B), my self-critic can switch me into a submissive role when I am entering a situation with people or during the conversation. For instance, if my self-critic says, "you're a fraud, you're talking rubbish, and everyone can see it", then it is likely to switch on a physical response in me that tones down my words and drains the confidence from my contribution. I might keep my thoughts and opinions to a minimum; I might keep the conversation on safe and agreeable ground; I might even appease and flatter the other person or people – to signal to them that I am not a threat. In doing so I am reducing the likelihood of drawing an opposing view or switching on competitive roles and feelings. What's happening here is that the internal competitive process in my own mind (my self-critical attacking) is preventing an external competitive process with others. A critic-initiated controlled explosion.

The self-critic can also help me with the final aspect (C), which is the challenge of having anger naturally switching on in my body, but also needing to keep that emotion contained – safely 'in house'. Of course, emotional activation involves energy – i.e. electromagnetic vibration frequencies in the atoms of our central nervous system. (No Charlie, don't start – you already said the physics lesson was over!) This energy creation is crucial to activating the bodily arousal required for protective responses (fight-or-flight). So where does this energy go? It cannot be routed into the fight-or-flight response that it was designed for. But nor can we expect it to simply disappear (and defy the laws of physics). The energy needs to be routed somewhere else *internally*. At the physical level, the energy needs to either be discharged somewhere else within the body or be held/contained in the body until it is safe to be *externally* discharged. (More on 'containment vessels' in the bomb squad equipment section, Chapter 5). At the psychological level, the self-critic can provide a suitable target – a home for the angry emotional energy.

"You fucking idiot piece of shit, waste of space"

Even just saying and typing that sentence gave me a little wave of energy release. Like all *controlled explosions*, there is a trade-off between the harm created (the self-inflicted explosion) and the harm averted. So here, the harm created to your mental well-being by angrily calling yourself a "*fucking idiot piece of shit*" is a worthwhile trade for the possible harm of being angry and creating a competitive situation with another person. Of course, the relative weightings of cost-vs-benefit in this trade will be influenced by previous experiences of other people. If I have experienced others as being hostile, attacking, and harmful in the past, then the controlled explosion of self-attack will be more favourable. In addition, there is the evolutionary context of our brain, which for many millions of years has primed us to err on the side of caution (*better safe than sorry*). The self-critical discharge of angry energy is the safer option here.

Self-submission as training rehearsal for future threats

Another way of looking at this self-critic (the **SUBMITTER**) is to also consider its possible role in preparing us for future threats. Every protection system needs training, rehearsals, and test-runs to check that everything works okay. And it's no different to the bomb squad. Eliciting a submissive response in us is something that has to be practised to ensure it will work properly when we need it for *real*. Without rehearsals, there would be a major risk of us being utterly overwhelmed or floored when a real threat arises. The self-critic offers us an opportunity to practise and train our body for protective, submissive responses. Even if there is no real threat or danger to me right now in my environment, there could be threats in the future. How will I know that my body will respond effectively to these future threats unless I've done a few test-runs?

> *Make sure you weave your parachute every day, rather than leave it to the time you have to jump out of the plane.*
>
> (Jon Kabat-Zinn)

For a training session to be most effective, the internally generated *simulation* of a threat has to be a fairly accurate replica of the (worst) real threat. It must be believable. The whole point of the training simulation is to elicit a *genuine* bodily response, to test that this response is working ok. We cannot risk the danger of being overwhelmed and demobilised by something far bigger and scarier than we've ever rehearsed. It would be no good if the self-critic was tasked with saying, "oh, you are a silly sausage"!

To simulate (and prepare for) real life threats, the self-critic must be experienced as a genuinely threatening entity. The ideal way to achieve this is to base the prototype of our self-critic on some of the real people or characters that we have learnt to associate with threat. This might be a scary authoritarian teacher from back in our school days. It might be a critical parent, or it might be a fictional character from a fairytale, movie, or story. For any chance of adequate simulation and preparatory training, the self-critic has to represent something that has become logged in our memory associations with dominance, power, fear, and threat.

A predictive processing account of self-criticism

In Chapter 1, in the section, *Our brain's relationship with reality*, we were introduced to the *Predictive Processing* model [7]. In this influential cognitive neuroscience model, we learnt that our perception of reality is not the objective reality per se, but rather a hypothesis or prediction of what we *expect to* see. So, what I am perceiving in this moment is not what is happening in front of me, but a hypothesis generated by my brain, based on my previous predictions and prediction errors from similar moments in the past – more like a prototype or template. So just to quickly orientate ourselves as to what this means exactly, let's consider an example: imagine I am walking along a beach one evening. As I walk along, my brain will be creating a prediction about the types of sensory events I might encounter while on the beach. In other words, my brain will be generating its own sensory information to predict what's about to happen. It will then compare these predicted sensory signals with the actual sensory signals from the world, and if there is a difference – a prediction error – its hypothesis templates will be updated for the next encounter.

As noted previously, this is a very efficient way of perceiving the world. If my predictions are accurate, I can carry on without using up too much of my energy resources. If there is a discrepancy, however, this will quickly stand out and I can allocate resources to minimising that discrepancy. I can do this in two ways: either by *perception* (changing my template to make a better prediction) or by *action* (changing the world to bring it more into line with my prediction). So, if we took our central theme of controlled explosions and looked at this through the lens of *Predictive Processing*, could it be that some of our *controlled explosions* are themselves a way of correcting a discrepancy? Some *controlled explosions* are perceptual (they elicit emotional and physical arousal in our bodies) and some are behavioural (they elicit actions to change something in the world). The common theme that connects all types is that they are protective, in that they function to avert some predicted harm.

According to the *Predictive Processing* framework, our past experiences are always an active component within our current perception of the world, and our brain is always doing things (perceptually or behaviourally) to minimise its uncertainty or prediction error. When it comes to situations of possible threat, our brain (as we have seen in Chapter 1) reserves the right to activate a particularly strong bias in our perception of the world. The accuracy of its predictions (and size of its prediction errors) become less important. Our brain's threat-bias will favour a perception that is most likely to keep us safe and protected in this moment. If survival is at stake, our brain will select a prediction, based on our past experiences and past predictions, that favours survival over accuracy.

We don't see reality. We only see what was useful to see in the past.

(Beau Lotto [5])

It's likely that we each have a handful of highly significant 'threat situation' templates in our brain; threat models from which we can select to shape our future threat perceptions. The prototype of a critic (a hostile other) will be an important one of these, because we'll need this close at hand to select in situations of threat from other people. However, the overall template will be comprised of not just the hostile critic alone, but also the experience of receiving hostility. It is the whole scene that our brain needs to model, so there are two aspects: both a threat-giver (the critic) and a threat-receiver. The critical part is *creating* the threat simulation, and the body is *responding to* this threat.

These two parts are simultaneously activated – they are two sides of the same coin. Cause and effect. Our predictive brain will select this whole scene as a *cause-and-effect* template. The same will be true for how our brain has predicted, processed, and stored previous memories. So, when I was mentioning before about the 'critic' prototype (which might be linked to memories of teachers, parents, fairytale monsters, and so on), we can expand this prototype to include the memories of all the emotions and bodily responses we experienced too. So, it is not just the critic that is switching on, it is the whole scene of threat stimulus *and* response.

What comes first? The critic or the submissive action?

The question of what comes first – the self-critical attack or the submissive action, is something Tobyn Bell and I addressed in our 2025 paper [11]. In summary, we suggested that both cause-and-effect sequences could be possible:

1   Self-attacking → threat response is switched on
    or
2   Threat response is switched on → brain selects a self-attacking perception

Although our brain might have initially formed the predictive model to fit the experience of receiving hostility from a person and then activating a submissive response, the way it is stored and triggered in our brain is more likely to be all bundled together as one. Remember, according to *Predictive Processing*, our perception in this moment is a constructed template, largely using memory, so the sequence of which comes first and second doesn't matter. This means that my 'threat-giving-and-receiving' template could be switched on either by receiving a threat from someone, or equally by a submissive sensation in my body. Both would need a predictive model. The templates are there to make predictions about the sensory information in my environment, but also about my own emotional and bodily states too. (This is the difference between exteroception and interoception.) In the latter case, my nervous system would be detecting the bodily state first, which is saying "I am feeling afraid, therefore there must be something to be afraid of", which then activates the template of 'the critic'.

One last thing to consider, before we meet the fifth and final member of this unit, is the possible function a critic may serve in providing an orientation to a source of threat. The critic itself is acting as a source. The alternative, if no critic were present, would be uncertainty – there may be an unspecified fear sensation in the body with no 'home' and no direction or orientation in which to mobilise action. The presence of a critic provides a source, and a clear set of directions for protective movement and action.

DISSOCIATOR: to create a dissociative response

This bomb squad member has the job of shutting down, exiling, or containing parts of our mind for safety and protection. These kinds of *controlled explosions* are some of the most forceful that our brain's protection system uses. This type of self-critic – our inner dissociation-maker – is only really called upon in extreme circumstances when the presence and awareness of a certain feeling, emotion, or need may carry a risk to us. The part of our experience that is deemed 'risky' essentially needs to be distanced and removed from our awareness. In some circumstances, it might be quite a targeted explosion to exile one part, but other circumstances might require segregation and isolation of multiple parts.

So under what circumstances might it be risky to experience a feeling or need? I described one example earlier where feeling anger might be risky. Anger may bring forward an action where we may confront or challenge another person, and that could in turn attract a strong retaliation from this person. If this other person is far stronger and more powerful than us, then this could put us in great danger. Aside from the immediate danger of attracting harm, there may be other dangers with anger in terms of social acceptability and social position. In some situations, anger could get us into trouble with our social group. It could result in us being sent to prison or in some other way shamed or rejected by our community. We might be seen as a less desirable person, which is also a major threat to us. This is the threat of whether we are socially accepted or rejected. Whether or not we belong in a group.

Our sense of the social acceptability of emotions will be influenced by messages we have received from our upbringing, including from our parents and communities. There are often strong cultural and religious attitudes towards a particular emotion or emotions. There are also social stereotypes to do with things like our gender, skin colour, and race that play a role in what needs we are expected to have and what emotions we are expected to feel or not feel. The internal relationships we have with different parts of ourselves is complex.

If we have learned that anger is bad, or we are in a situation where anger is risky, we may need to find a way of distancing ourselves from the experience of anger. One way is to try and contain the emotional energy in our body somehow, so that it is held and braced in our muscles, and does not lead to actions. Another way is that we can try to cut the emotions off at source by removing the reasons for even feeling these emotions in the first place. The body-holding option will be explored more in Chapter 5 when we discuss 'containment vessels'. In terms of removing the *reasons* for emotions, what I am referring to is how we might attempt to disown or deny some of our basic needs.

If we could convince ourselves that we don't *need* love and belonging, then we won't feel sad or angry when we don't receive it. If we convince ourselves that we are a bad or unlovable person, then we won't feel so angry when people treat us badly or neglect us. This way we can attempt to keep the anger switched off, or at least not visible and not expressed to the outside world. But rather than channelling anger into confronting or fighting the other person, we might instead attack the part of us that is causing our inner conflict or pain. So the anger is not switched off per se, it is just redirected towards ourselves and towards our own vulnerabilities. For example, rather than attacking my parent for not meeting my needs, I might attack myself for having a need. If I no longer had a need, then the conflict would be resolved, and the anger towards the parent would no longer be there. In other words, we want to destroy the part of us that is causing us pain, rather than attack the 'other', which could be dangerous.

HARM CREATED: *Attack or disown the 'needy' part of me*

HARM AVERTED: *The fear of being disowned if I showed anger about my unmet needs*

Attacking our own needs – such as our need for love and care – or for recognition and respect – is not always about managing anger. It might also be about managing sadness too. For example, it can help us to remove, postpone, or delay the experience of a loss. If we didn't have a need in the first place, then there is no loss. No unmet need → no yearning and longing. No painful grieving of this loss. So sometimes these self-attacks (or attacks on our needs) are about avoiding the pain linked to sadness, grieving, and loss. Again, part of this is avoiding the uncomfortable feeling itself, and part of this is about avoiding the action and behaviour that could be mobilised from having this feeling. In the same way that anger might come with 'risky' actions like confrontation and challenge, sadness might come with risky actions like crying and sobbing and making ourselves small, weak, and vulnerable.

HARM CREATED: *Attack or disown the 'needy' part of me*

HARM AVERTED: *The fear of being sad, vulnerable, weak, and small*

If we have a need to be liked, our self-critic might specifically attack that need ("no-one likes you"). If we have a need to be respected and admired, the self-critic might attack that need ("you're useless and worthless"). If we have sexual feelings or needs, the self-critic attacks these ("you're a slut"). If we have a need to feel cared for and looked after, the critic might attack that need ("you're pathetic"; "stop acting like a baby"). The *controlled explosions* used by this self-critic – the **DISSOCIATOR** – are designed to suppress and split off these needs and emotions, and *as a result*, the actions that would risk – or hinder our survival of – a far greater threat.

The splitting process might require some force

To achieve dissociation, this member of the bomb squad might need to generate a fair amount of forceful energy towards the part that needs 'removing'. This may even require quite a violent controlled explosion attack. Just as we thought the **SUBMITTER** self-critic wouldn't have much success by saying "you silly sausage", neither would the **DISSOCIATOR** self-critic have much success by asking an emotion to "kindly do us a favour and keep quiet". These are high-threat, high-stake situations we are talking about. There is no time for a polite conversation. The emotions themselves will be firing up with plenty of energy of their own, wanting to get involved to do their protective jobs, so the dissociation-maker's energy will need to not just counter that, but overpower it. The **DISSOCIATOR** will need to be strong, forceful, and direct. The goal is removal. And fast.

It is no wonder, therefore, why some of the self-critics I have encountered in my therapy practice can be so harsh and abusive. They are direct and blunt, going straight to the heart of people's greatest insecurities, shame, and fears. This is particularly true of those who have experienced terrible traumas and tragedies in their lives. These are the people who have had to use dissociation as a survival strategy in extreme situations. The extremity of the situations has warranted the intensity and forcefulness of their controlled explosions.

Body triggers of self-attacking

In the previous section on the **SUBMITTER** self-critic, we learnt that the sequence of cause-and-effect can occur both ways: (i), where a self-critical attack leads to a protective body state; and (ii), where a protective body state leads to the perception of self-critical attack. The same is true for the **DISSO-CIATOR**, in that the body states of dissociation may trigger the perception of an internal self-attacker. So what kinds of body states are associated with dissociation? When we are trying to suppress an emotion, such as anger, our body might need to assume a kind of 'brace' position. So this means a particular pattern of muscles in our body will need to be tensed and tightened (for example, maybe around our jaw, shoulders, or fists). Suppressing different emotions might have slightly different body profiles (for example, involving areas across the chest or 'lumps' in the throat). There are also more generalised body profiles we can switch on to brace the body for a wider emotional suppression. These are more like a full-body detachment, numbing, or even a full 'freeze' or 'shut-down' response. The freeze response is designed to put our whole body into a state of immobility. We can still see the external world, but we can't feel or move our body.

Most animals are equipped with a freeze response, and with abilities to shut down and immobilise their body movement. It's a key part of an evolved survival response. In humans, we are basically the same, except that many of the 'newer' brain functions we have evolved, such as our human perceptual, cognitive, self-monitoring systems also get tied up in, and recruited into serving, these protective processes. We don't know this for sure, but we doubt that other animals have hostile self-critics that accompany their dissociation. But as humans, we do. Our perceptual and conceptual systems are constantly working in parallel to our sensory, emotion, and motor systems. Making predictions, best guesses, hallucinations – whatever our brain can generate to help us stay alive.

Preventing re-traumatisation

When a trauma occurs in a person's life, the first task is to survive the immediate situation. To stay alive. If fight and flight are not possible, the person will automatically resort to submit, dissociate, shut down, or freeze. If they do successfully survive this situation, the second task is to make sure that re-traumatisation doesn't occur. This means avoiding anything that might carry a risk of re-traumatisation: a risk of being in that situation again; a risk of re-experiencing the traumatic pain. The brain essentially goes into a mode of trying to regulate how much emotion and pain can be allowed to enter the person's awareness, and when. The **DISSOCIATOR** is acting a bit like a gatekeeper or a night-club bouncer, saying what is and what's not allowed to come in. This is how it protects the person. Part of that is about splitting off needs, as we have already seen. Needs carry a risk of pain, so they're not allowed in. But what other sorts of things might carry risk and not be allowed? What about hopes and dreams? These could be quite risky too. Getting too optimistic about the future might run the risk that it could all suddenly be taken away. What about talents? Potentials? The **DISSOCIATOR** self-critic, in its attempts to protect the person, may shut many of these down too. This may lead to the sabotage of opportunities, connections, and interests.

> [The inner protector will] *do all it can to prevent* (what it believes will be*) potential re-traumatisation. In doing so, it becomes an unwitting and violent inner persecutor.*
>
> (Donald Kalsched, clinical psychologist [38])

In terms of the bomb squad, this is like a controlled explosion that has been initiated but then continues to have cascading and perpetuating explosive effects. The initial explosion required strength and force (rightfully so, essential in fact). But the ongoing effects of this forceful explosion can continue to create ripples that devastate a person's life and can really deny them their future potential, fulfilment, and happiness for many years to come. People can become trapped in a cycle of self-criticism, shame, dissociation, and depression.

But then the big question is *"What can we do about this?" "How can we approach this?" "Do we approach this by exploding the explosion?"*

"Criticising the critic?" "Attacking the attacker?" It's complicated, because remember the attacker is a protector. Of course we do want to reduce harm, but how can we do this wisely, in a way that doesn't *increase* harm? Although it may be tempting, if we just simply started attacking the self-critic, we could easily compound and escalate the explosions. It's like repeatedly firing more and more bombs at the same target. This would keep the threat active and keep the perceptual and body systems suspended in patterns of conflict. The person would now be fighting threats each day, new threats arising from their own minds. Their survival strategies themselves would become new sources of threat. This compounding battle upon battle could ultimately lead people further and further away from, and losing touch with, the *original* threat, which was of course the trauma.

This is where understanding the concept of *controlled explosions* is so vital. The bomb squad are not the enemy; they are there for a reason. We can try to understand them and use their *controlled explosions* to show us the route towards what we really need. We can trace the function of these explosions, these self-sabotaging behaviours, back to their original source, to the original fears and traumas that initiated the protective processes in the first place. For trauma survivors, the **HARM AVERTED** in our template is typically the underlying fear of re-traumatisation, and the **HARM CREATED** is anything to avoid that.

It is these underlying perceived, predicted fears that have been driving these processes all along. It is these underlying fears that desperately need our compassion and care.

In Chapter 6 we will be exploring ways of approaching our inner controllers. But before then, we still have a whole new bomb squad unit to meet, the Self-Harm Unit.

Chapter 4

Self-Harm Unit

Controlled explosions that can harm us physically

Chapter summary

This chapter explores controlled explosions that cause us physical harm. Sometimes this is directly self-inflicted, and sometimes it's through eliciting harm from others. We will consider some different versions of this, some of which are day-to-day occurrences, and others that are linked to more serious mental health concerns and support needs. In line with the overall theme of this book, the focus will be the function and role of the Self-Harm Unit. We will consider how even these more severe forms of self-generated harm might still be functioning in ways to protect for other (bigger) potential threats. This chapter will link in with some of the clinical understandings and formulations of addiction, eating difficulties, and self-injury, whilst also recognising how many of these patterns also play out as milder, day-to-day versions, throughout the population, without ever reaching 'clinical' thresholds for distress or needs.

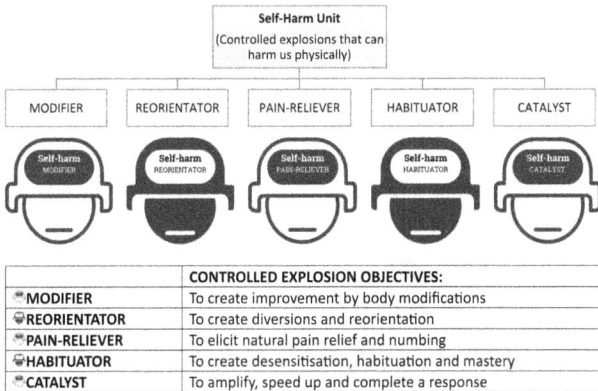

	CONTROLLED EXPLOSION OBJECTIVES:
MODIFIER	To create improvement by body modifications
REORIENTATOR	To create diversions and reorientation
PAIN-RELIEVER	To elicit natural pain relief and numbing
HABITUATOR	To create desensitisation, habituation and mastery
CATALYST	To amplify, speed up and complete a response

Members, roles, and objectives of the Self-Harm Unit

DOI: 10.4324/9781003559924-7

The term *self-harm* is usually used to describe when we inflict pain and damage on our own body. This often refers to when we deliberately cause external injuries to ourselves, such as cutting, burning, scratching, picking, or biting. However, it can also refer to causing ourselves internal injury, such as putting toxic amounts of drugs or alcohol into our body, or by depriving ourselves and our bodies of basic needs, for example, depriving ourselves of food (as with fasting), sleep, or social contact. Another form of self-harm is when we deliberately put ourselves in a situation where harm is highly likely to occur. So, for example, we might participate in unsafe sex, or we might provoke a person into becoming angry or aggressive towards us. We might voluntarily offer ourselves (and our bodies) to be dominated or controlled by another person. In the doodle, I have written out some of these examples in a (pretty grim) word cloud.

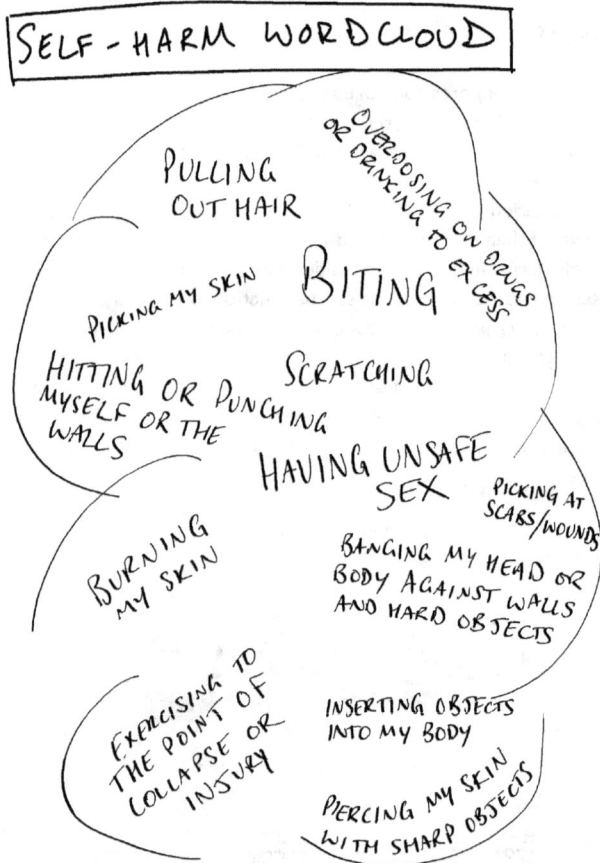

SELF - HARM WORD CLOUD

PULLING OUT HAIR

OVERDOSING ON DRINKING TO DRUGS OR EXCESS

PICKING MY SKIN   BITING

HITTING OR PUNCHING MYSELF OR THE WALLS   SCRATCHING

HAVING UNSAFE SEX   PICKING AT SCABS/WOUNDS

BURNING MY SKIN   BANGING MY HEAD OR BODY AGAINST WALLS AND HARD OBJECTS

EXERCISING TO THE POINT OF COLLAPSE OR INJURY   INSERTING OBJECTS INTO MY BODY

PIERCING MY SKIN WITH SHARP OBJECTS

DOODLE: "Self-harm word cloud"

In this chapter we will explore each of these self-harming behaviours as being the kinds of strategies used by five different members of the Self-Harm Unit.

MODIFIER: to create improvement by body modifications

Have you ever caused physical harm or pain to your own body to better yourself in some way? It might be that you have pushed your body to its limits as part of an intensive exercise regime. You may have heard a fitness coach say things like: "feel that burning sensation", "push through the pain", and "we need to break the muscle down to build it back stronger". Indeed, the old exercising mantra 'no pain, no gain' still gets used in many different life domains beyond fitness and sport. In a workplace context, for example, a 'no pain, no gain' mentality might mean working extra hours, never taking sick days, and making other personal sacrifices to succeed and progress in your career.

When it comes to emotional and mental health, we are often encouraged to push ourselves outside of our comfort zone, to face our fears, to build our resilience. We might have learned that 'exposure' to our uncomfortable feelings can help us overcome fear and anxiety. Many of us will have also tried fasting, which is restricting our food intake for periods (hours or days) at a time. If so, we may also have experienced some of the harmful impacts of nutritional deficiency on our bodies, such as headaches, dizziness, or stomach pain. In these examples, exposing ourselves to some forms of physical and emotional pain may be motivated by self-improvement. There are of course important differences between discomfort and pain, and it may be that the wiser coaches, advisors, and therapists out there would be the ones helping you to distinguish these, and to recognise that pain would be a signal to stop.

Cosmetic alterations for self-improvement

Sometimes we might seek to change things about our body with the intention to improve our physical appearance. With our body hair, we might regularly shave, pluck, and cut. With our skin, we might scrub, peel, and exfoliate. We might have cosmetic procedures to change the shape of certain body parts – whether its surgical operations to our breasts, face, hair, nose, stomach, thighs, and so on, or the non-surgical use of chemical injections, peels, and lasers. The important thing here is *intention*. Typically, the intention is to improve something for us, whether physically (such as our appearance) or psychologically (such as our confidence or well-being.). Although, on the face of it, these acts of 'cutting off' or 'injecting in' are highly invasive and forceful towards the body parts themselves, the overall motivation would still be considered self-improving. Hence, this could fall within a broader definition of *controlled explosions*, i.e. self-initiated harm with the intention of helping in some other way.

So how can we differentiate whether an act of interfering with or re-configuring the body is self-improving or self-harming? Is it as simple as asking, "what is your intention and motivation?" And if the intention is self-improving, does it matter if this is about physical self-improvement, or an improvement that's entirely psychological? (*"The reason I want this cosmetic procedure is to boost my self-confidence and improve my emotional well-being"*). You can see how it's a complicated job for surgeons, psychologists, and other health professionals to disentangle people's intentions. Often the task is to assess whether this is coming from a place of *genuine* self-care, or whether it may be driven by underlying insecurities and fears. In many cases, there's a bit of both, as can be revealed by something as simple as how the question is phrased: instead of asking "what is your intention for having this procedure?", you could ask "what would be your greatest fear if you weren't able to have this procedure?". The second question is much more likely to open some of the underlying fears that we all have as humans, linked to basic needs, such as social acceptance and belonging. This brings us even closer towards understanding how this falls within our framework of *controlled explosions*:

HARM CREATED: *Choosing to cause harm and pain by reconfiguring my body*

HARM AVERTED: *Fear of being unattractive, undesirable, and socially isolated*

It becomes even trickier when we consider things like body dysmorphic disorder (BDD), which is a clinical condition where someone strongly perceives and believes that they have a defect in their physical appearance, even though this perception and belief is not shared by others. So, if this person said that they had an intention to improve their physical appearance, do we conclude that this is not a *genuine* intention? This is clearly a complicated area, and our aim in this book is not to make judgements about what is real or not, and to distinguish between the experiences of those in clinical settings compared to the rest of the population. In fact, this book takes a 'continuum' view, in that understanding day-to-day forms of mental suffering can be extended into understanding more severe versions of suffering that we see in clinical settings. And vice versa; that clinical conditions like eating disorders and BDD can help us better understand our daily struggles, particularly the self-inflicted explosions and self-sabotaging harms that our brains can bring upon ourselves.

Body piercings and tattoos

Other forms of body modification include tattoos and body piercings, which are very common, have been around for centuries, and are becoming increasingly popular in modern culture. The motivational drivers for altering our bodies in this way are multiple and varied, ranging from beauty, art, and fashion, to expressing self-identity and individuality. Other motivators might be for establishing group affiliations/commitments, for protesting against parents or society, for spiritual and cultural traditions, for reclaiming the body, for sexual reasons, or for testing out physical endurance (for a full review, see the article by Wohlrab and colleagues in the journal, *Body Image* [39]). From this list, some motivators might align to more of the protective functions that we have explored in this book (for example, where it creates a sense of control or mastery), while many are not related to any such emotional function or context. There are of course people who can develop quite impulsive and addictive relationships to modifying their body, and others who can take it to quite risky levels. So, it may be worth keeping an eye on how that relationship develops over time. Piercing and tattooing may start becoming more closely linked to emotional functions over time, even if that was not initially the case. This is where there may be some crossing of the boundaries with addictions, as well as self-injury, which is the topic we come to next.

REORIENTATOR: to create diversions and reorientation

Many people who physically self-injure report that it helps them to release a build-up of emotional tension, which already indicates a controlled explosion (one harm created to avert or lessen another harm). But why does creating harm to the body reduce emotional distress? One possibility is that it creates a diversion, in that our attention and awareness is immediately orientated to the 'new' (physical) harm, making us less aware or less preoccupied by the previous distress. This may provide a welcome break or temporary respite from our suffering.

Orientation to self-injury (such as cutting, burning, scratching, picking, or biting)

A self-inflicted physical injury, such as cutting through the skin, is more than just a diversion and distraction away from the original (emotional) suffering. It is an entirely different type of harm as well. For starters, the cutting action is within the person's control. This means that an orientation to self-injury provides some degree of certainty. The person can control the timings (start, duration, stop), the depth, the length, as well as the whole environmental context in which the cutting takes place. Many self-harmers have a ritual around the cutting; a sequence of actions, which provides further predictability and certainty to the harm.

These factors may be preferable to the volatile nature of emotional suffering, which often feels out-of-control. This is because emotional and mental health suffering is often caused by a complex web of factors (biological, psychological, social, environmental), so there is not such an obvious cause-and-effect model to makes sense of it. There is no start and stop either, so the fear is that this suffering could persist for hours, days, months. Evolution has given us a brain that craves certainty. In the words of Beau Lotto, "Certainty meant life. Uncertainty meant death" [5]. So when we are struggling with emotional and uncertain suffering, it would be our **REORIENTATOR** that creates a controlled explosion to divert our attention towards a new harm. This new harm is more predictable and therefore feels more manageable and controllable.

There are more day-to-day examples of self-inflicted harms and pain that we may be familiar with. For example, a family member recently told me that she always bites her thumb really hard before having her flu and Covid vaccinations. Many people talk about picking their skin or biting their fingernails when feeling nervous. (For lots of us, skin picking and nail biting may have started off as a mini-controlled explosion but then developed into a habit over time.) The phrase "biting your lip" refers to suppressing an emotion, suggesting that it may be rooted in some kind of strategy for emotional avoidance or control. Recently on holiday, I noticed that when I had been bitten by mosquitos, I would (over)scratch the bites on my legs – I mean *really* going for them. And as I was driving my fingernails deep into my legs, I wondered whether perhaps I was more comfortable with the certainty of my own *self-generated* harm than with the mildly irritating (and yet still out-of-control) harm from the mosquito!

In a fascinating study by de Berker and colleagues in London, they found that the stress-levels of their participants were higher with the *uncertainty* of not knowing if they would receive an electric shock, compared to the certainty of knowing they definitely would or definitely wouldn't [40]. Does biting our thumb before an injection create a pain *diversion*? Does it create a pain *certainty* that's more in our control? Does it create a *brace response* in me that controls my reaction to the jab? Maybe it's a bit of all three. Perhaps one reason why we are so desperate to avoid uncertain harms and pains in the world is that we might not be able to control our reactions to them. And if we can't control our reactions, then this could lead to a cascading effect of yet more harms happening. For example, if I am not in control and braced before an injection, is there a danger that I might let out a massive yelp? And if so, might I then have the social embarrassment of being looked at by the other hundred people in the vaccination centre? Probably safest just to control the explosion.

Food, substances, and chemicals

Self-harm by putting substances and chemicals into our bodies is also some-thing that we have choice over and control. So again, even though these sub-stances may be very harmful to our body, this might seem like the least-worst option, where the alternative is unrelenting and out-of-control suffering. We can control food intake to harm our body (too much or too little). We can also choose whether to introduce chemicals like drugs and alcohol into our system – what, when, where, and how much. Of course, as the psychoactive effects of these substances start to influence our decision making, we might start to lose some control over our decisions. So, although we may have been in control of the decision to start, we may have less control over the decision to stop. In that sense, this could be seen as *a controlled way of losing control*, which sounds contradictory, but actually could be a highly effective controlled explosion – a controlled entry into a state that frees you from the worry of having to make further choices.

Another aspect we can control with food and chemicals is the type of re-sponse that we are eliciting in our bodies. For example, our bodily sensations and perceptions will be very different if we eat a tub of caramel ice cream com-pared to a spicy hot chilli dish. Also with drugs, we might choose a narcotic drug like heroin that produces sedative effects, or we might choose a stimulant like cocaine. Being able to manipulate the sensations and effects gives us cer-tainty and predictability, which is what we humans are programmed to need.

There are various ways that we can create *controlled explosions* in our body using substances. For example, we can add a substance into our body that elicits:

- a **threat** *(stress/protection)* response – which either diverts attention away from the emotion or overwhelms it
- a **drive** *(pleasure/reward)* response – which either diverts attention away from the emotion or overwhelms it
- a **soothing** *(calm/comfort)* response – which either diverts attention away from the emotion or down-regulates it.

These strategies correspond to Paul Gilbert's three systems model [29, 41], which is a helpful framework used in *Compassion Focused Therapy* to map out the different systems we have for organising our emotions and emo-tion regulation according to their evolutionary function. An example of some foods that might elicit a stress response are those high in added sugars or caffeine (tapping our cortisol/adrenaline). For pleasure and reward responses, we might go for junk food and those high in carbohydrates (our dopamine). And for soothing, we might opt for a nice creamy cheese or a comforting tub of dairy ice cream (our opioids). These are day-to-day food choices we are all making. Of course, for recreational drug-users, there are not dissimilar choices being made (albeit slightly more illegal). *"Do I want to feel more alert, more joyful, or more relaxed?"* *"Do I want a drug that activates my adrenaline, dopamine or opioid receptors?"*

We take strong things to produce strong reactions

If we are struggling with an intense emotion, our **REORIENTATOR** might need to create an explosion in our body that is equally intense. If the explosion is not strong enough, it is unlikely to be successful in either diverting attention away, or overwhelming/overriding the emotion. A packet of plain 'Ready Salted' crisps might not have the same impact as a packet of 'Salt and Vinegar'! A glass of beer might not have the same impact as a tequila shot. So depending on the level of harm that we are trying to avert, we might need to adjust the level of harm (strength, toxicity) created by the substance. There are many similarities here to what we were saying in the previous chapter about needing a strong (and hostile) self-critic to elicit strong protective reactions.

As many drug-users will know, there is the issue of developing tolerance. Over time, we become more habituated to the effects of a substance. The strong effects become less strong, and so higher quantities or potencies of the drug are needed to recreate the same strength. The same is true with food and diet as well. If food is being used to override or soothe our uncomfortable feelings, then this can lead to overeating. *"I need to eat the whole packet of chocolate biscuits now to feel the same effect that I used to feel with just one or two."*

Restricting food

We have so far been focusing on the effects of adding food and substances into our bodies. However, the restricting or depriving of food is another type of controlled explosion that can be used by the Self-Harm Unit. This time the harm comes from removing the basic nutrients and energy fuel source that our bodies need to function. As with the addition of food, the restriction of food can elicit different emotional responses for people. Some might feel a sense of reward or achievement for being able to conquer their eating urges, or by achieving a particular body shape or weight. The sense of power and control we can feel (over our body) might be very satisfying and gratifying to us, especially if we are feeling a lack of control in other areas of life. This can be quite addictive.

For others, it might be the numbing of feelings that is protective. No food, no calories, no energy. There is only one way this can go – towards a general quietening or blunting of sensory signals around the body. The problems are still there, but the perceptions and signals being received by the brain are toned down. The diminishing energy reserves are having to be directed to even more basic needs, such as heart-beating and breathing. This process, common in anorexia nervosa, is one of the most dangerous forms of self-inflicted harm that we explore in this book. As the energy drains out of our system, we start losing the cognitive capacity to change, or perhaps even notice, the dangerous direction. Our controlled explosion, even though it may have been initially protective for us, has now rendered us utterly powerless to even look after ourselves and our precious life.

As we have said many times throughout this book, while *controlled explosions* may be functional (protective) and understandable in certain contexts, it is important that we in no way underestimate the utterly devastating and life-threatening harm that they can create for us. Remember, I am writing this book to raise awareness of *controlled explosions* so that we can become aware of them and choose what to do with them. This will be the focus of Chapter 6, and there are worksheets in Appendix 3 that might help you work through any of the *controlled explosions* present in your own life. However, if you're feeling confused about something you've read in this book, or you're not sure what to do, please speak to someone. This could be a trusted friend, a family member, or a therapist. I know it sometimes feels hard to speak, and we don't always know the words to say, but please start the conversation anyway and just give it time. The words will eventually follow, and the understandings will start to fall into place. In Appendix 5, I have also provided a list of some websites, books, and resources that could help you identify what additional needs you may have for help and support.

Purging

Purging is typically associated with a form of purification or cleansing – removing 'bad' things from our bodies – i.e. things that we perceive may be causing us harm. In the context of skincare, for example, the intention of purging is generally to remove toxins, impurities, and to shed dead skin cells. In the context of food and eating, purging refers to the self-initiated, and often forceful, removal of matter from inside our body. This might be through self-enforced vomiting or misusing substances like laxatives and diuretics as a way of inducing diarrhoea. Again, the motivations behind purging could be multiple. The intention might be to help yourself to feel better by removing something harmful that you've ingested, or if you've ingested excessive amounts. We might, for example, force ourselves to vomit if we've drunk too much alcohol – we want to get the toxic substance out of our body to help us feel better (now or in the morning). Sometimes we might force ourselves to vomit if we have eaten too much food and feel uncomfortable or ashamed about the amount we've eaten. We might worry that something we ate is not good for us, and it's *'better out than in'*. At the severe (clinical) end of this continuum is bulimia, where people can enter into a distressing pattern of binge eating and purging. My Balanced Minds colleague, Ken Goss, is one of the leading experts in this field and has written a self-help book to support people caught in these cycles [42], which is included on the resource list in Appendix 5.

Although the motivation may be to help through cleansing and purifying, there are of course harms, which is why purging is another good example of controlled explosion used by the Self-Harm Unit. Forcing ourselves to vomit can be very harmful to our bodies and can destabilise the balance of our natural organ functions and chemical processes. For example, it can propel stomach acids into our throat and mouth, which were supposed to be digesting food in our stomach. Bulimia, of course, can be devastating for a person's mental and physical health, and is often associated with significant amounts of shame and self-criticism.

> **HARM CREATED:** *Forceful, self-induced vomiting*

> **HARM AVERTED:** *Uncomfortable feeling of having 'bad' or excessive matter in my body*

Eliciting harm from other people

Have you ever intentionally started an argument or provoked an angry response in someone? Or maybe you've seen a film where a highly distressed character starts a fight? I'm imagining a classic movie scene where we see the emotional turmoil of a character who is maybe going through a major breakup, bereavement, or loss, sitting there slouched at the bar ordering whisky after whisky. And after a few strong drinks have gone down, they turn round and pick a fight with the big muscly guy playing pool with his big muscly friends.

> *"Oi you, come over here you big lump of muscly so and so ..."*
> (That is not an actual film quote, it's one I made up – but you get the picture.)

So what's going on here? Is this a version of self-harm where we are getting other people to do the harming to us, rather than ourselves? The Self-Harm Unit can create explosions from the outside-in. They can provoke reactions in other people (emotional or physical).

There are subtle differences here between the jobs of the **REORIENTA-TOR** and the **CATALYST** (who we will meet later). The **REORIENTATOR** uses the environment to create a diversion away from the emotional pain that we are experiencing, whereas the **CATALYST** uses the environment to amplify the emotional pain, to make it bigger, louder, and more pronounced, so that it can be expressed, discharged, and completed. So, coming back to our movie character drinking whisky at the bar. If the character was feeling sad, lonely, and ashamed, his **REORIENTATOR** might start a fight to divert attention away from these emotions (e.g., sadness, shame) or to overwhelm/ override them with a new emotion (e.g., anger). It has summoned up a more pressing matter. As we will see, the job of the **CATALYST** would be more to step in if the character was feeling angry, but the anger needed to come out in some way. So the **CATALYST** would start the fight to create a home and outlet for the anger. They are both *controlled explosions*, but with a slightly different objective.

Creating threat in the external world to reorientate from our internal world

As well as eliciting reactions in other people, the Self-Harm Unit can also create environments and situations in which harm is likely to occur. For example, think about somebody who engages in dangerous activities, like extreme sports or unsafe sex. Sometimes we might do these things more recklessly than other times, for example, if we were really pushing the limits in a 'thrill-seeking' sport, or doing it more haphazardly, without care, and without the right safety equipment. We might also enter ourselves into social situations where we are likely to encounter threat, maybe entering an online discussion forum or a social media thread where we know there are strong and hostile views being expressed. Sometimes we might seek out extreme political views that are diametrically opposed to our own. We might post something that we know is controversial, in a place where we know it will be read by people who are easily outraged. (In the UK, we have a phrase for this: "to put the cat amongst the pigeons".)

Many of us will be familiar with the compulsion to drive our car faster when we are upset or emotionally distressed (either in our own lives, or again from the movies). When we are feeling overwhelming emotions, we might consume riskier quantities of alcohol, drugs, or food. We might wander round the streets at night. We might seek out more extreme, intense, or risky sexual encounters with people we've never met, or start searching for equivalent images and videos online. We might spend large amounts of money on consuming and shopping (impulse buying), or risk more of our money on bets and gambling. We might even feel like doing something illegal or criminal, thereby risking trouble with our community or the Police.

Why are we edging ourselves closer to danger? Is this a way of managing an overwhelming emotion? There are many ways that we can engineer our world to give us strong threat signals, and in turn these threat signals will activate our flight-or-flight reactions. From the perspective of this book, therefore, it may be that we are using our world as a kind of controlled explosion. We are creating threats in the world (towards ourselves) to orientate and mobilise our threat emotions and responses. Like starting a fight, these risky behaviours and self-generated threats may be designed to grab our attention and override whatever it was we were feeling before. From this perspective, perhaps it's understandable why we are drawn to riskier things when we're feeling stronger emotions. Stronger emotions feel more overwhelming and out of control. They are disorientating, and so there may be more need for a controlled explosion. A diversion that grabs our attention. A reorientation. A sense of focus, certainty, and clarity of what we need to do. It may be that we are creating risk and danger in the external world to reorientate our awareness away from our internal world.

There are similarities here with the **CHAOS-CREATOR** from the Self-Sabotage Unit; however, with the Self-Harm Unit it is actually *harmful* what we are bringing our way, and therefore even more important that we notice when this is happening in our lives. If we are intentionally inflicting harmful experiences upon ourselves to avert something else (like an overwhelming feeling), then this is really something we should know about. With knowledge and awareness comes wisdom and confidence to make different choices. *"Am I making the wisest choice here?" "It may be understandable why I am drawn towards this risky behaviour, but now I can see what's driving it, is there an opportunity to help the emotion in some other way?" "Is there a way of helping the emotion to feel less overwhelming for me?" "Can I slow down and take time with it?" "Or if I'm not (yet) ready to address the emotion directly, is there a less harmful strategy or behaviour I can use in the meantime until I am ready?"*

PAIN-RELIEVER: to elicit natural pain relief and numbing

This unit member uses self-harm to release the body's natural defences against harm and pain. This is very similar to the angle we took when we were trying to understand the various roles of the bomb squad's Self-Criticism Unit. Members of that unit were characterised not by the nature of the criticism they direct towards us, but by the response they elicit in us; for example, the **SUBMITTER** (a submission-maker) and the **DISSOCIATOR** (a dissociation-maker). So what is the equivalent for the Self-Harm Unit? Physical self-harm can also create submissive and dissociative responses, so some of the previous chapter will also apply here. However, due to the physical nature of the harm we will focus more closely on the body's chemical responses.

Creating pain for the (subsequent) pain relief

The body responds to self-injuries such as cuts and burns firstly with pain and then with the experience of pain relief. The brain's natural pain-relievers (called endorphins) are triggered, and once released, their job is to block the pain receptors in our brain. So, by creating a targeted physical pain in our body, we may experience a more generalised pain-relieving experience that blocks the perception of both physical and emotional pain. Creating pain is creating pain relief. This type of controlled explosion is illustrated in the doodle. The self-harm is therefore creating an altered sensation for the individual, a kind of numbing and detachment from sensory perceptions.

> **HARM CREATED:** *Controlled physical pain. Body's natural pain-relief systems initiated*

> **HARM AVERTED**: *Emotional pain, suffering, torment that feels persistent and out of control*

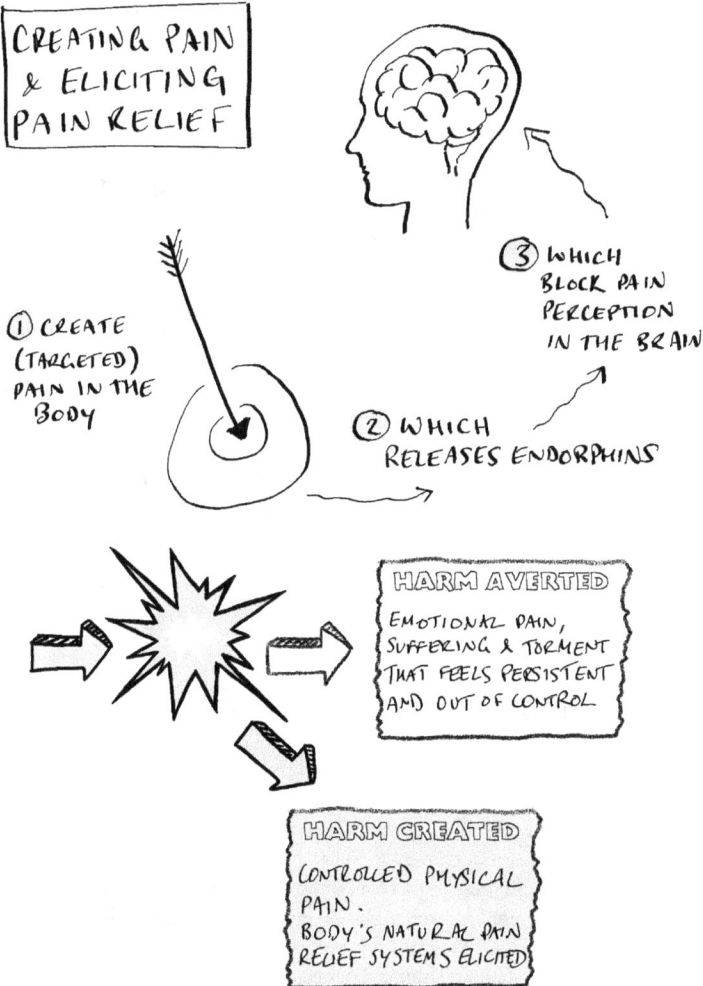

DOODLE: "Creating pain and eliciting pain relief"

Other forms of self-harm can produce similar effects. A numbing effect is known to occur through the restriction of food and starving the body. This is one of the functions reported by anorexia patients, who are caught in a terrible and dangerous cycle of controlled starvation, self-attacking, and emotional numbing. We can also elicit a pain-relief reaction by hitting ourselves or punching our fist against the wall. Pulling our hair can be incredibly painful but can then create quite a pleasant tingling sensation once the initial pain has passed. Each case is an example of creating pain for the subsequent relief. As bodybuilders and sports people might know, a similar effect can occur during strenuous exercise as well.

The runner's high

After a long period of running and muscle workout, many runners report experiencing an exquisite, blissful feeling. This is often reported to become possible only after a good 4 or 5 miles of intense running. Even though the runner's muscles have been strained, utterly worn out, and exhausted, there is a beautiful moment of calm and euphoria where their bodies just feel like they are gliding along. (I am imagining this is how Neo in *The Matrix* feels when he first experiences his superhuman abilities.) For that moment, which may be brief or could even last up to an hour, the runner feels like they have entered into a 'flow state', where they have absolute mastery over their body and their sport. It is not clear the exact chemical composition of this state, but most likely a release of endorphins or endocannabinoids (the same system activated by the THC in cannabis), or a combination of the two. So, this is a naturally occurring neurochemical response to intense bodily strain and stress, which is not only pain-relieving, but also pleasurable and euphoric. There is a sense of calm, as well as mastery over our bodies and our emotions.

Flow states

The term 'flow states' is used to describe mental states where somebody is fully immersed and focused on a task or activity. They are fully in the zone, skilfully absorbed in the moment of what they are doing. The chatter of the analytical, self-reflective mind is switched off (you know, the *"how am I doing"*, *"what does this mean"*, *"what do other people think of me"*, and so on). None of that. We are just present, absorbed, in control, and 'at one' with our activity. Even time is suspended. We can experience flow states with any activity, from sports, to mindfulness, to book-reading, to video-gaming, to creating art. While these are generally associated with positive experiences that boost our mental health and well-being, it may be that some self-harming acts are an attempt to create something similar. There can be a combination of pain-relief from sensations and emotions, a dissociation from negative thoughts, whilst also being in a heightened state of body mastery and control.

It is complicated to think about the intention here because, on the one hand, the intention is to harm my body. So, on the face of it, this is coming from a desire to hurt and cause harm. However, if you asked the person what their intention is, they would probably say "to take away the pain", "to give me a break from suffering", or "to release my endorphins to give me a numbing or even a pleasant feeling". So, is this a self-harming motivation or a self-caring motivation? Or both? This really highlights the importance of understanding *controlled explosions*, and hence the reason why I really wanted to try and write this all down for you in a book! The point is 'it's complicated', and yes it can be both. We can intentionally cause harm to ourselves in order to care for ourselves! There is a harm created, *and* a harm averted. It's both. And so, before we take a rigid position of whether this is good or bad (we like certainty, remember!), can we instead hold both the goods and the bads, the pros and the cons, in mind together. There are two harms. And if I could go to the balcony and look back at both of these harms, what would I do to help? From this third perspective (me on the balcony), what do I understand about these two parts? One part of me wants to create a harm and the other part wants to protect me from a harm. How can I help these two parts work out a wise solution? More on this in Chapter 6.

HABITUATOR: to create priming, habituation and mastery

In Chapter 1, I presented the example of how a vaccination works. The vaccine primes our immune system. It gives our immune system the opportunity to *get used to* the experience of having a virus in the body and how to deal with that.

> **HARM CREATED:** *Add virus or antigen to mimic infection and to prime immune response*

> **HARM AVERTED:** *Having a body that is unprepared to recognise and fight a disease*

This unit member, the **HABITUATOR** has the job of creating *controlled explosions* in order to train and prepare our body for threat by becoming *accustomed* to the presence of threat. This is a bit like the fire alarm tests that you get in a building – a threat-rehearsal of sorts. You are intentionally activating the protective response that may be required – in this case, a building evacuation. There are a number of ways that the **HABITUATOR** goes about training and rehearsing our body's protective responses, but let's start with an example from sport.

Contact sports are those where a player is required to make physical contact with another player or players. Boxing or wrestling, for example, or martial arts.

Rugby is a good example of a team contact sport, and so is NFL (American football). If you went along to a rugby match and watched the players warming up before kick-off, you would see them going through various drills of whacking their chests and shoulders against pads, in what are called 'contact drills'. They are habituating their bodies for the contacts that will come in the match. The body is able to practise its tensing and bracing patterns for hits (both given and received).

Desensitisation occurs when we arrive at a place in our training when we can no longer even feel the hits or the pain. We have become fully habituated or acclimatised. Nothing can hurt us now. This might feel that we have conquered or mastered the pain, and can now go into battle (or sports match) with great confidence and no fear of getting hurt.

In this section we are interested in *self-harm* versions of this. Where we might be harming our bodies as a form of training – to create readiness and preparation.

Harming our body to build strength and resilience

We may be familiar with the concept of harming bodies, in some contexts, as a display of strength. Many tribal societies, for example, have used initiations and rituals for thousands of years, to prove status or readiness, or to act as a transition (a rite of passage) into adulthood. These might involve difficult or painful ordeals of physical suffering for the person to prove themselves and demonstrate that they are ready. Although these formal initiation ceremonies have mostly died out in modern societies, there are still some signs of similar things going on (in a less formal, ritualised way).

In my younger days, this was certainly the case, particularly as a teenager at school and then as a student. Being able to drink huge amounts of alcohol, or take a large quantity of drugs, was seen by many as an opportunity to display their adulthood or strength: *"I can handle it"*, *"I can drink you under the table"*, *"I am the last one standing"*, *"I am the 'king of the bongs'"*, *"my body can take the hits"*. We might take pride in building up our body's tolerance levels, and this in turn may give us some reward and social capital, for example, attracting admiring comments from others, like, *"wow, your body is like a machine!"* We might relish the process of building up our tolerance levels over time, and actively pursue this as a goal. We might like testing how much strength and quantity we can handle and then proudly bang our shot-glass on the table after we've knocked back our tequila. We relish the chorus of cheers that ring out if we've successfully managed to 'down' our beer in one. If you go to a cricket match in the UK, you occasionally witness an entire crowd of 25,000 spectators all cheering together when someone gets up in the stands to down their pint (to be fair, there might have not been much else to cheer about in the 4 or 5 days passed of the match so far!).

When I mentioned body piercings and tattoos at the start of this chapter, I cited Wohlrab's literature review which identified 'testing physical endurance' as one of the motivators reported by people [39]. Finding ways of bashing and bruising our body, from the inside and out, can make us feel strong – so that we can tolerate and endure the pain.

Some psychological parallels to this process were mentioned in the section about the **CHAOS-CREATOR**, with one of the functions being to develop mastery over chaos, uncertainty and out-of-control feelings. Here, we have the physical equivalent – where creating physical harms may function as a route to developing mastery over bodily stress and pain.

Habituation and desensitisation following a harmful experience

In addition to the physical 'strength display' versions, there might be other versions of **HABITUATOR** functions that arise directly following trauma and difficult life experiences. If, for example, our body has been physically or sexually harmed in the past by another person, we might develop ways of preparing our bodies for the feared eventuality that this could happen again. Again, this would be linked to the imperative to avoid re-traumatisation. Some ways that people might do this include harming their bodies to create numbness, detachment, or dissociation. This is a way of desensitising the body's feelings and sensations. Sexual abuse survivors often learn to treat and relate to their bodies like 'objects'. This is protective because objectifying their bodies would make the experience less painful if abuse were to happen again. Many develop strong hatred and disgust towards their bodies, which may be part of the same process of distancing and disowning. Self-injury, drugs, and depriving of food are other ways that abuse survivors may attempt to desensitise their bodies to physical pain. This may sometimes involve repeatedly training the 'brace' or 'numb' response in certain body locations where the physical harm has occurred. Sometimes this might be about training the whole body to be able to totally detach and become disconnected from awareness altogether. Developing the *total* body detachment ability would be one sure way to prevent the possibility of re-experiencing the overwhelming pain of bodily trauma in the future.

CATALYST: to amplify, speed up, and complete a response

This member of the Self-Harm Unit creates controlled explosions that amplify, exaggerate, and ignite a response that it feels needs to happen. The **CATALYST** might achieve this by influencing our environment in a way that would be sure to bring forward the emotion and response. It might elicit emotional or bodily harm from the outside-in. There was a member of the Self-Criticism Unit we met earlier, the **DISCHARGER**, who was similarly concerned in how to address the pent-up or incomplete emotional cycles held in our bodies. That bomb squad member relied on the self-critical (self-to-self) relationship to unblock the emotions and get them flowing again around the system. The **CATALYST**, on the other hand, uses other-to-self and world-to-self relationships to ignite and speed up these flows. It engineers situations and interactions that will create 'a home' for emotional expression.

This time, our starting point for meeting this member and building an understanding of its function is probably not quite what you'd expect. We will start with a sausage cooking on the barbecue! First of all, did you know that in the UK we call our sausages 'bangers'? (as in 'bangers and mash'). You may already have known that, but do you know why? Apparently it's because in the First World War, they used to put fillers, such as water, into meat (due to food shortages and restrictions). So, when you cooked a sausage, it expanded quickly and often exploded! Nowadays, not much seems to have changed, for me at least. I don't know if it's just my cooking, or the type of sausages I buy, but this also seems to be exactly what happens when I cook sausages on the barbecue, especially when the temperature from the charcoal is very hot. The sausage starts forming steam bubbles in their outer layer, which begin expanding rapidly. I can see they're getting bigger and bigger, and before they have a chance to explode all over the place, I perform a *controlled explosion*: I carefully prick the sausage with a knife. This means the steam can escape through the little hole, and the danger is averted.

This is similar to the **CATALYST**. It creates a controlled outlet for the building-up emotion. Something from the outside that can come along and speed up and release the tension. The **CATALYST** craves closure. It doesn't like having loose ends or incomplete emotional processes. It doesn't want to leave sausage-expansion to find out its own destiny. It wants to get the job done, now, and get it over with. It's not about suppression, avoidance, or distraction, like some of the other bomb squad members we've met along the way. It's about getting the response done quicker.

Amplification

Sometimes getting the job done requires amplification. This was not the case for my sausages; they seemed to be racing nicely towards an explosion anyway. In that scenario, amplification would have involved me turning up the heat or lowering the sausages closer to the charcoal. In other situations, it might be a bit uncertain as to whether or not an explosion will occur, so the **CATALYST** might just come along and resolve that uncertainty for us by giving us a clear signal. For example, consider a situation where you might have a hunch that another person is angry with you. You're not entirely sure, but they have been a little bit quiet today, and bit 'off' with you, and they didn't laugh at your joke earlier. You feel that something might be up. It could be totally unrelated to you, of course (they might have something else on their mind), but you're not sure. You are finding it hard not knowing. The more you worry and ruminate about it, the more you start building up a predicted scenario in your mind where this person could be *really* angry at you and may suddenly turn around and explode – as in, start raging and yelling at you. This is where our **CATALYST** might step in. The uncertainty is becoming unbearable, so just to achieve closure on this situation you might behave in a way that brings forward this person's anger. You might *stir up the hornet's nest.*

Idiom: *stir up a hornet's nest*

Meaning: *to create trouble; to cause an uproar; to cause an upheaval; a commotion which possibly ends in anger and frustration*
(Source: www.theidioms.com)

Creating 'a home' for an emotion

When we perceive an emotion brewing in us, as opposed to in another person, this unit member might create a context in which this emotion can be expressed. If the emotion brewing in *us* was anger, the hornet's nest might also work as the controlled explosion. We behave in a way that stirs up the anger in them. They then express their anger towards us. And we've got an ideal scenario in which to be angry back at them! We've created 'a home' for our anger – a world where it can run free. In the **REORIENTATOR** section we imagined a movie scene where someone drinking whisky at the bar provokes a fight with the big muscly guy playing pool. In this instance, the person was creating a distraction *to not* feel a particular emotion. In the case of the **CATALYST**, the function would be the opposite. Picking a fight with the big guy holding a pool cue would be *to* feel the emotion. To bring forward the anger that is brewing and needs to flow. This is about releasing the build-up of tension.

There could be many other ways that people create homes for their anger. Not just with people, but also with environments and situations. Some are healthier than others. This might be one motivator behind why some people take up contact sports, for example, or join the army and go to war. These are situations that will involve competing, and therefore opportunities to exercise and express their competitive emotions. They might join a debating club. (I am reminded of the classic Monty Python comedy sketch, where a man goes to the *Argument Clinic* to pay for an argument.)

There might be other places that offer similar opportunities and homes, such as an activist or protest group who are fighting for justice, or for human rights, or for the environment. Of course, engaging with these things is, in themselves, not at all problematic, and very important in democratic societies. But what we are talking about here is the controlled explosion version – when the motivation is linked to the expression of anger, and not to the topic or concern of the group itself. For example, we are thinking about the person who joins a protest outside a government building, not because they care about the cause itself, but because they are looking for a home – any home – for their anger. They might show up at every protest, for every cause. Every time there might be a riot, they are there. This is about them, and these situations are their catalysts for their own *controlled explosions*.

Some believe that a similar thing could be happening on social media, particularly to try and understand the behaviour of so-called 'trolls'. If you have unprocessed anger brewing up inside your body, and that anger is looking for a 'home', the internet will welcome you with open arms! There are limitless opportunities to start arguments, provoke people, make insults. Anyone, anywhere, anytime, can get into 'virtual' fights from the comfort of their own homes. And they can do so anonymously without even having to deal with any negative consequences afterwards. In that sense, the internet has given us a highly controlled type of controlled explosion. We can be having a raging exchange with someone one minute, and the next minute be logged off and watering the house plants. Other common ways that people find homes for their anger are through action movies and video games that involved fighting and shooting. The **CATALYST** is relishing the future when even more immersive versions of these will come to our homes, as virtual reality technology becomes more available and accessible to us all. We may be able to create a *home* for our anger, both metaphorically and literally.

A race to the bottom (perhaps rock bottom)

Wanting closure and completion for emotional tension is all very well. But most things in life are not that simple, and getting to the end of a process usually takes time, with twists and turns along the way. The **CATALYST** doesn't like twists and turns. The impatience and hastiness of this unit member, and its preference for direct (over wiggly) paths often lead to the premature foreclosure of a problem. Sometimes this process is very dramatic. And sometimes the **CATALYST** races us straight to the most extreme and very worst place.

In Chapter 1, when introducing the concept of controlled explosions as a protective strategy, I gave the example of "eating all the doughnuts and beating myself up". This is classic **CATALYST** work. Let's set the scene: We are walking back home one day, after a busy shift in our office job. It's Monday, so we started off tired, and we've been at our desk all day in front of the computer. Nothing particularly unusual about that, but we're feeling exhausted. We have also been struggling with our food choices recently. We've been trying to watch our weight, trying to make more healthy choices, and trying to be a bit more careful with snacks at work and during the week. We've been trying to move away from the unhealthier options, like chocolate bars and crisps. So we're walking home, past a supermarket, and we fancy a little snack as a 'pick me up'. The first thing we see, next to the entrance, is a shelf full of freshly made custard doughnuts. *"Perfect"*, we think. *"One of those would be big enough to hit the spot. It'll give me a satisfying first bite, and then an oozy creamy goodness will soon follow."* It doesn't look too unhealthy either. It's been freshly made today here in the store, so that must be a good thing. It's not glazed. Good. And it's definitely not crisps or chocolate. Excellent. The only downside, we're thinking, is that they only come in a pack of five – *"That's annoying, so I'll have to just eat one now and keep the other four in my bag"*. We then have a counter-thought: *"Actually, maybe five is quite good, because that means I'll have one for each day of this week."* And that would mean a whole week where we've managed to avoid crisps and chocolate. Great.

We eat one. *"Wow. That hit the spot. That was just as good as I imagined. I could eat another one of them."* Simply having this thought, *"I could eat another"*, sets off an internal tug-of-war in our mind. One part saying, *"no don't"* and another part saying, *"but I could"*. Back and forth, back and forth. As the tension rises from this internal debate, and the corresponding stress responses become more active in our body, the two parts get a bit more intense in their role and debating style. The part saying *"no don't"* is now becoming quite critical – *"You're a silly idiot with no will power. Grow up"*. And this provokes a defensive reaction in the other part. The other part doesn't particularly care about the doughnuts anymore, it is now just reacting defensively to being belittled and being told to grow up. A power-play has started – one part (*"no don't"*) is taking the role of an authority figure or parent, and the other part is stepping into the role of a rebellious child that doesn't want to be told what to do. The threat system is online, there is anxious tension, rumination. It's hard to tell where this will go. Uncertainty about where this will end … Send in the bomb squad.

The **CATALYST**'s job is to speed up and get this conflict to its conclusion. Over and done with. That means to hurry the debate along to its 'furthest' or 'worst' point. The most extreme version, the endpoint – the version we would eventually reach if we allowed this conflict to play out all the way through to its natural conclusion. The **CATALYST** wants that 'natural conclusion' endpoint, but it wants it here and it wants it now.

HARM CREATED: *I eat all the doughnuts and beat myself up to get it over and done with*

HARM AVERTED: *Indefinite rumination, uncertainty, and anxious tension*

This controlled explosion has essentially brought forward the predicted (future) endpoint, and made it happen now. The endpoint, or most extreme version, of the rebellious child's position is to eat the whole pack of five doughnuts. The endpoint, or most extreme version, of the authority figure's position is to punish the child. Then it's over. Finished.

This might help us start to see, therefore, how this kind of controlled explosion has the potential to catalyse quite a dramatic 'race to the bottom'. The further away and more extreme we predict the endpoint to be, the more dramatic the explosion needed to get us there. To get closure. What if the *only* endpoint we can imagine is being punished? Perhaps that was what we experienced a lot as a child, and so that's why our brain has learnt to predict it. Would our brain catalyse punishment from another person for the sake of closure?

HARM CREATED: *I'll take the beating and the pain now*

HARM AVERTED: *Avoid sitting with the uncertainty of will I/won't I be punished*

What if the only endpoint we can imagine is *rock* bottom? If that's the case, then that's likely to be where the **CATALYST** is setting its sights on. If left to its own devices, that's where it would want to take us for certainty and closure. Anything less would still be flavoured with unsettling and uncomfortable feelings of uncertainty. *"Am I there yet?" "Is there more to come?"*

This need for speed and closure may therefore result in quite dramatic acts of self-sabotage and self-harm. If we are struggling with alcohol, rather than food choices, we might drink the full bottle of vodka to get it over with. We might take ourselves into extreme and dangerous places with our health and bodyweight – places which ultimately take decisions and choices out of our hands. For example, we might find ourselves in a place where we have put on 20 kilograms, and we drink all day. We might also keep ourselves isolated from other people in the process. Other people can complicate things for us – they say things, they might question us and try to stop us. We worry that this will only keep us in uncertainty and indecision for longer. Delaying the inevitable. Our **CATALYST** can't bear uncertainty and delay. It wants to find the place of certainty – of no more decisions and choices. And that may be rock bottom.

Is rock bottom the endpoint or the beginning?

One of the things I am very interested in, in my work as a therapist and researcher in mental health, is the concept of post-traumatic growth. One of my favourite books I've read on the subject is *When You're Falling, Dive* by Mark Matousek [43]. This book is full of inspiring stories of people who have used their pain to transform their lives in a positive way. Many of the people had reached terrible points in their lives – rock bottom – and come back stronger, wiser, and with a purpose that far transcends anything they had felt before in life.

For me an interesting question, therefore, when it comes to *controlled explosions*, is whether something like the **CATALYST** is fast-tracking a *destructive* process or the initiation of a *healing* process? Perhaps it is both, and the choice is very much yours. Once you've hit this wall, what do you do next? In Chapter 6, we will be addressing questions like these when we think about how we can approach our *controlled explosions*. What you may not realise yet is that once you've identified your *controlled explosions*, you get to write the script about what happens next. It's up to you whether you write a setback story or a *comeback* story.

Chapter 5

Equipment/kit

Equipment used to support controlled explosions

Chapter summary

This chapter explores some of the additional psychological structures and processes that can help to support the bomb squad with their controlled explosions. We will look at 'containment vessels' as what our brain uses to hold or isolate certain emotions that are deemed harmful, as well as 'disrupters' and 're-mote detonators' which are what our brain can utilise to trigger controlled explosions. The 'remote detonators' may come into play when particularly high or forceful levels of explosion are required. Here it might be more effective to create an external (remote) source from which to trigger the impact, than an internal one. This chapter will therefore touch on experiences such as voice-hearing, which are experienced as intrusions coming from outside of our minds. There will be some insights from clinical populations and literature here but, again, as we have done throughout this book, these experiences will be considered on a continuum throughout the whole population – things that all of our brains can generate.

Police bomb squads use all sorts of interesting kit, gadgets, and tools to go about their heroic and risky work. This equipment is to help them protect people in as safe and effective way as possible. For example, they walk around in giant bomb suits and helmets to protect themselves. They also have sophisticated X-ray machines to assess the internal mechanisms of bombs, how to disable them, and to determine exactly where to target their controlled explosions, and how much force to use. They have equipment to prevent explosions, to contain them, or indeed to initiate them. Some equipment is designed

DOI: 10.4324/9781003559924-8

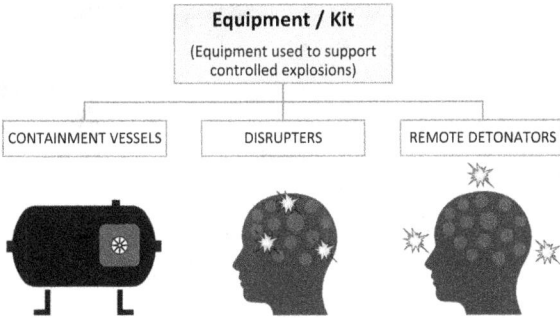

	CONTROLLED EXPLOSION USES:
◉CONTAINMENT VESSELS	To hold and contain emotional activation
◉DISRUPTERS	To disrupt processes that could lead to harm
◉REMOTE DETONATORS	To initiate impact from an external location

Equipment/kit and their uses

to disrupt and prevent a harmful explosion from occurring in the first place. Some is designed to create a safe distance and separation between an explosion and its controller. Some is designed to create a safe contained environment for explosions to occur. In this chapter, we will consider all these various functions as we take a rummage through the kit room at Bomb Squad HQ.

Containment vessels: to hold and contain emotional activation

One of the most effective ways to mitigate the harm of a large blast is to surround it with a very strong container. A 'Total Containment Vessel' (TCV) is a useful bit of kit for any bomb squad, with its fully enclosed, gas-tight inner chamber and its fortified walls that can withstand maximum blast pressure. A containment vessel can be used to deal with many threats, such as bombs and hazardous materials, in a controlled environment. This protects people and the environment from all sorts of things like flying fragments, gases, and other omissions from an out-of-control blast. In my research for this book, I must confess I did spend a few (too many) hours watching YouTube videos of TCVs in action (recall the **PROCRASTINATOR** in Chapter 2!) In these videos, the bomb squad chief shouts: "*Fire in the Hole!*" before pressing the red button and detonating the blast. Here is a little six-step diagram that I created, which is not supposed to be an accurate technical portrayal of a TCV, but rather my own highly simplified interpretation for this book! Essentially: hatch is opened; explosive device is inserted; hatch is closed; boom; hatch is opened again to release the gases.

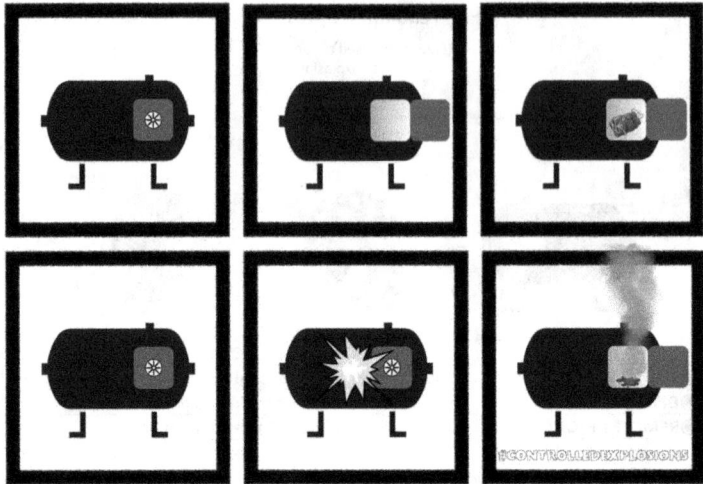

(My interpretation of) a Total Containment Vessel (TCV)

So how does this relate to our internal processes as humans?

Our body may need to contain a sensory-emotional trigger from becoming an action

There are times when our body needs to contain an explosion, for example, to prevent it from getting out and causing problems in the world. Many of us will be familiar with the experience of having to hold back our tears, or to bite our lips. Perhaps an emotion–action sequence has been initiated in our body but cannot be allowed to complete. It may be too risky, for instance, for us to physically follow through with the muscular motions and actions that are triggered, especially if these actions could put us in danger or lead to negative consequences. So instead, we have to contain and store this energy build-up. To keep it 'in house'. And this is when we need to use our internal containment vessels.

In Chapter 3, we learnt about some of the occasions where an energy sequence might be activated in our bodies but where the cycle cannot complete. This is when we were meeting the **DISCHARGER**, whose job it is to release and complete these built-up energy stores. In Chapter 4, the **CATALYST** was also in the business of getting emotions out. But before any release can happen, there is of course the containment and storage stage itself. The TCV footage that I watched on YouTube shows how this equipment is usually mounted on trailers, so can be easily moved around. This is important because it might not be safe to release the smoke and gases in the immediate location of the threat. It might be safer to drive a few miles down the road, or a hundred miles into the desert, before it is safe to open the hatch. The same is true for the (emotional) containment vessels in our bodies. If our boss has annoyed us during a meeting at work, we might have to bite our lip until the meeting is over. Then once we have safely left the building, and are walking back home through the park, we might choose that moment to call our colleague and have a massive rant down the phone.

Our bodies typically store this energy in the regions and muscles in which the emotion would have been expressed (if it were allowed and safe). So, for example, if you were angry but had to hold back the anger expression, you might store up some tension in areas like your jaw (grinding/clenching) or in your fists. If you felt sad, but had to hold yourself back from crying, you might be storing some heaviness in your chest and shoulders. If you had to suppress these kinds of emotions repeatedly and frequently, and were greatly restricted in your opportunities for discharge, then your body may have had to develop some longer-term storage solutions. For example, you might have developed a generalised internal numbing system. A way of masking or suppressing the emotional and sensory signals. There may be a chronic build-up of stress and tension in parts of your body, which may eventually find their own way of being expressed in the form of physical pain or physical health symptoms.

When using a containment vessel, remember to open the hatch afterwards

Containment vessels are not supposed to be permanent storage solutions. They are vital for temporarily holding some energy for us, at least long enough until it is safe to be moved or released. Bear in mind that, unlike TCVs, the human containment vessel is not made out of fortified steel, it is simply flesh, muscle, and bones. So there is also an energy cost in keeping our body tensed in the kind of 'brace' position that is required for emotional containment. The longer we leave our bodies in this braced holding pattern, the more energy resources we use, and the more tired, exhausted, and depleted we become. Hence why it is so important to remember to open the hatch from time-to-time; to release and discharge the tension. Having said that, however, there may be some situations where it could serve us to self-initiate a stress response, and to then contain it for a prolonged period. One example could be if we are doing some kind of endurance training or if we are trying to develop tolerance and mastery over pain.

An inner fortress where we can encounter pain safely, and with mastery

Like all the other muscles in our body, we do benefit from keeping our 'brace' muscles exercised and trained. At various points in this book, I have highlighted the role of controlled explosions in the context of training and rehearsing for real threats in the world. One example is when we introduced the **HABITUATOR** in Chapter 4, and at other times, it has been in relation to exercising our threat 'muscle' and developing tolerance and mastery over difficult emotions. Here, the containment vessels can really come into play. If, for example, it is important for us to prepare for painful things in the world – things that will involve pain tolerance, resilience, and endurance – then it may serve us to have some practice with holding and tolerating emotional tension in our bodies. Training our bodies to get used to the feeling of prolonged tension and stress may have helped our ancestors to take more risks, to courageously venture further out into uncertain terrains, knowing that if the worst happened, they would have a chance of dealing with it.

It is clearly all about balance, however. Endurance training through experiencing some conflict, distress, and pain *does* build resilience. However, too much or too many of these experiences can start to have the opposite effect, and lead to a downward spiral. Perpetually having to endure and hold stress in our bodies is ultimately going to weaken and deplete us, rendering us less able to courageously go out into the uncertain world. To be able to master pain is likely to involve finding the 'just right' amount of usage of our containment vessels.

There may also be times where we need to brace ourselves for the anticipation of imminent harm. So, in this instance, we would need to self-activate the emotion, hold it in our containment vessel, and wait for the expected harm to arrive. And at that point of harm arrival, we will already be energised, charged, and ready. Take your mind back to the rugby players doing their 'contact drills' before the match. Hence, if we are predicting a future threat, our brain might create a 'simulated' threat first to get the brace system online and ready for the 'real' threat. For the rugby player, these would be the contact pads made from high-density foam and PVC material, designed to mimic and simulate the contact that is about to come later from a (very large) human's shoulder. For the person who fears being attacked or harmed by other people, these would be the kinds of self-attack or self-harm that we have been exploring in this book. The containment vessel allows the bomb squad to practise these self-attacking and self-harming explosions. It's an inner arena in which we can safely encounter pain and practise our resilience and coping.

Do we need to discharge excess energy before we can rest?

In the mornings, I often go outside for a run with my dog, Dora, along the coast. It usually takes about half an hour. (Definitely not long enough to experience the 'runner's high' from the previous chapter, which remains ever illusive for me!). When we get back home, I typically get ready for a day of work while Dora gets ready to have a nice long sleep. However, I have noticed an interesting thing about her sleep-preparation ritual. When we come in through the door, she rushes straight inside and has a short intensive burst of play-fighting with the rug. She strongly shakes the rug in her mouth, growling at it, and running full pelt around the room. This whole episode only lasts for about 30 seconds, before she casually wanders off to find a place to lie down and nap. So, what is this all about? She is not really a growly or barky dog. She's generally pretty laid back. This is very uncharacteristic of her, and something that seems uniquely related, as far as I can tell, to the context of returning from a run. It makes me wonder if this is something to do with a discharge of excess energy. Perhaps her body has initiated some muscular, motor energy to prime her for running, but for whatever reason (probably because I'm too slow for her liking!) there is still an excess amount that needs releasing before she can go to sleep. Is her **CATALYST** speeding something up for her to get closure?

Can you think of any parallels of this in your life? Are there any times when you have an excess amount of energy after doing something? I was trying to think of parallels in my life too, but after I exercise, I generally want to sit down. The last thing I want to do is rush around at full pelt, shouting and yelling! But then again, I am not going to sleep straight afterwards like my dog. My body will be awake for at least another 14 hours. I'll be seeing clients in my therapy clinic, having meetings, doing teaching, and speaking to people about mental health. Then the kids will get back from school, and so on and so on ... The run is only the start. My body could probably do with keeping some of its energy or at least releasing it more slowly and gradually as the day goes on. Something that I have noticed, however, is that if my anger has been activated by someone or something before my morning run, then I do sometimes notice myself cursing under my breath while running along. (Poor Dora!)

This also makes me think about some of the other behaviours that we touched on in Chapter 4 – things that we might be more likely to do when we're stressed, such as driving faster in our cars or acting in a slightly riskier way than normal. It is healthy to find ways to release; to give our body's containment vessel a bit of a rest. We have to discharge so that our nervous system can re-regulate. But where we may have to be careful is when we are using one controlled explosion help us deal with another controlled explosion – we could get caught in a bit of a self-destructive cycle. A healthy version would be to notice if we are holding tension in our body (one way, perhaps, is through mindfulness practice), and to intentionally give ourselves time, space, and care to fully feel what it is that we need to feel.

Disrupters: to disrupt processes that could lead to harm

Disrupters are used by bomb squads to disable a bomb. A disrupter is a carefully positioned device that can generate enough force to fire a projectile (such as water) at a precise target at an extremely high speed. The target may vary; for example, it may be the fuse (the initiator or precursor to a main explosion), the electronics, the power source, or some other component of the bomb that is necessary for it to detonate or explode. By taking a powerful, explosive shot at this specific target, the disrupter can disable or separate some key components of the bomb, which will prevent the main (more harmful) explosion from occurring.

> **HARM CREATED:** *An explosive shot fired to split or separate bomb parts*
>
> **HARM AVERTED:** *The whole bomb exploding*

Disrupters are very effective pieces of kit for disabling a bomb, but they do come with certain risks of their own. Firing a shot at a bomb is not something that you'd necessarily want to be standing too close to, even if you're wearing a full bomb suit. And the greater amount of force required for your shot, the more distance you might want to put between yourself and the impact area. This is where additional equipment comes in handy, such as remote detonators and remote-controlled robots. With these tools, bomb squad members can keep themselves at a safe distance, whilst operating a robot. The controlled explosion can be performed remotely. The robots are typically equipped with wheels, cameras and robotic arms, which enable them to achieve a precise, controlled and *external* firing of the disrupter shot. With the benefit of a remote location and distance, the intensity of the shot can now be increased. So, if the splitting of bomb components requires a very high degree of force, you would almost certainly want your remote detonators to be initiating these shots, not you.

In Chapter 3, on the topic of self-criticism, we learnt that our self-critics can take many shapes and forms, from milder forms of self-improvement monitoring, through self-blaming, self-disliking, to more intense forms of self-hating and self-attacking. Towards the end of Chapter 3, we met one member of the Self-Criticism Unit, the **DISSOCIATOR**, whose job it is to initiate a splitting process in our minds through quite hostile forms of self-criticism. We also noted that this splitting might require some force, which is why I would like to bring dissociation back into our discussion here. In the current chapter, we are considering some of the kit that is used to help generate controlled explosions, so it may be helpful to just quickly recap what we understand about the function of dissociation. Dissociation will help us to think a bit about disrupters and splitting, before we go on to consider situations where a 'remote' (external) detonator may be required for some of the more forceful types of dissociation.

Dissociation is an automatic and adaptive process that splits off unbearable parts of our experience. In the context of trauma, for example, our brains may have to disconnect some signals from entering our perceptual field. This may be particularly distressing emotions or sensory signals from our bodies. It may sometimes be a more generalised process, where many parts of our body signalling become disconnected from entering awareness. In these traumatic moments, if we were a 'whole' integrated self, it would be too unbearable. There would be too much sensory overload, and it would be very hard to function. We need a filter system, a way of separating out parts. A disrupter can be used by the bomb squad to break up the existing circuits and structure that comprise or awareness and sense of 'self'.

In an early article, published in 2011, I described another dissociative process whereby two important senses of our 'self', which are usually in sync with each other, become desynchronised. These are: our sense of *self in relation to the external world* and our *self in relation to the internal world* [44]. In that paper, I differentiated between two processing systems, conceptual and perceptual, although now I would probably further distinguish perceptual systems into 'exteroception' (perception of the external world) and 'interoception' (perception of our internal body states). Dissociation could be quite specific (for example, the compartmentalising of individual parts, emotions, needs) or a more generalised detachment between our perceptual systems. Either way, a disrupter is being used to break up some system or circuit in the brain. This is equivalent to how bomb squad disrupters target either a bomb component (such as the fuse), or a more general system (such as the electrical circuit or the power source).

HARM CREATED: *Dissociation to split up emotional or perceptual parts*

HARM AVERTED: *The whole system getting overwhelmed by threat signals and emotions*

Remote detonators: to initiate impact from an external location

There are certain situations when the type of explosion required cannot be adequately achieved by a bomb squad member alone. The bomb squad reside 'in house' – they are internally based; they are parts of us – and an internally experienced (self-to-self) harm or disruption can only be effective up to a certain extent. There are other times when we may need to experience an outside source of harm, i.e. coming from the external world. These may be quite extreme situations, for example when the magnitude of protective response required cannot be adequately generated from even the most hostile forms of self-attacking. This is when we may need to engineer an explosion coming to us from an outside source. I have already shared some examples of how we can self-sabotage by eliciting 'situations' in the external world (such as chaos creation), and examples of how we might elicit critical and hostile behaviours from other people towards us. In this section we will explore another example of controlled explosion, whereby our brain creates a perceptual *illusion* of something coming from the external world, when in fact it is being generated from inside our brain. This is why I have termed this section *remote detonators* – because the explosion is experienced as coming from an external (remote) location, even though it is internally operated.

For many years I have worked with people with a diagnosis of psychosis. These are people who often perceive threats from the outside world which are not perceived/perceivable by other people. A wonderful colleague and inspiration for my early work in this field, Isabel Clarke, uses the term "non-shared realties" [45]. These are experiences that are very real to the individual experiencer, but not to others, and they can take the form of either hallucinations or delusions. The hallucinations of people who receive psychosis-related diagnoses are often auditory – hearing voices that other people cannot hear. These voices can be very distressing for people because they are often directing criticism, threats, and hostility towards them, either through their words or emotional tones. Understanding the function of distressing voice-hearing was a major topic of my 2022 book, *Relating to Voices*, co-authored with another inspirational colleague, Eleanor Longden, who is herself a voice-hearer [14].

Hallucinations do not always come in an auditory (voice-hearing) form; they can also be perceived through other sensory modalities – for example, seeing visions, smelling smells, and so on – these perceptions can also signal the presence of threat (such as a hostile figure lurking in the shadows, or a smell of burning, or for those who have been sexually harmed, the threatening smell may be that of another person's sexual arousal). The delusional beliefs that people with psychosis report are also typically infused with themes of threat. Persecutory delusions (also called paranoia or paranoid beliefs) have indeed been characterised as threat-beliefs by one of the leading experts in the field, Daniel Freeman [46]. These delusions involve the perception or anticipation of danger that is developed into a conceptual belief system, story, or narrative that 'fits' or makes sense of the causes of a threat signal. So, for people with persecutory delusions, there may or may not be hallucinations involved. Sometimes a hallucination might contribute to the formation of a delusion, but at other times, we might perceive a hostile intention coming from people who do (physically) exist in the world. This could be anyone from powerful tech corporations and government agencies to someone's own family and friends. This is not a hallucination of sensory information; it is a hallucination of intentionality. The delusion is often an attempt to piece together a cause-and-effect story for the 'out there' that fits my sense of anticipation of being a recipient of hostility 'in here'.

The hallucinatory capacity of our brain is quite remarkable – the fact that our brain can trick us into perceiving threatening voices, people, intentions 'out there' is truly extraordinary and highly worthy of our time and attention on exploring and understanding why this happens. However, what is so tragic and inexcusable, in my opinion, has been our persistent and collective neglect of seeking to understand this important part of our human experience. Particularly in Western cultures, we have simply dismissed these experiences as symptoms of mental illness, and we have invented an elaborate system of categorising these into 'mental disorders' (schizophrenia, schizoaffective disorder, delusional disorder, and so on) which actively discourage us from exploring and understanding them further. It's a pathology. A symptom of X, Y, or Z [insert scary-sounding medical term]. And that's all we need to know. Let's instead focus all our collective efforts and multiple billions of dollars on developing treatments to get rid of this. We just shut these experiences down, and we encourage all experiencers to do the same. Imagine if one day in the future, we decided that human dreaming was an illness. We decide that all that nonsense taking place inside our brain as we sleep is all hallucination, and therefore a symptom of an ill or disordered brain. It's not real and must therefore be eradicated and banished from our brains immediately. It may sound crazy, but that's exactly what we've done with the corresponding experience that our brains create for us while we're awake.

So why might we have evolved a brain that can trick us in this way? Well, as with most brain processes, whether they are motivational, cognitive, emotional, or perceptual, the bottom line usually comes down to survival. Our brain is ultimately in the business of keeping us alive. Sometimes perceptual accuracy is a good thing for our survival. At other times, the time and energy resources required for achieving accuracy would be detrimental to survival. We need short cuts. We need best guesses. Sometimes we just need urgent mobilisation and action, and this might mean acting on only a vague hunch or gist of what might be going on. Perhaps sometimes we don't even have the slightest hunch of what is causing a threat – we just sense it – so it may be quite simply that *any* protective action will do, and in *any* direction.

Because perceiving an external threat is likely to elicit a more powerful protective action than perceiving an internal threat, it may have been useful for our brain to evolve a system of self-stimulation through hallucinating the presence of external threat. The British neuroscientist, Anil Seth, describes how even our experience of being a 'self' is itself a hallucination – a perceptual prediction that serves to regulate and control the interior of our body; ultimately, to stay alive [10]. Most of the time these functions are served well by the prediction that we are an integrated whole self (*"I am me"*, *"these are my own thoughts"*, *"this is my own body"*). However, under extreme circumstances, there may be times when this perceptual prediction of selfhood is *not* the most helpful thing for us. For example, there might be times where disconnecting from our embodied feelings and sensations might serve us better, such as if our body is being severely harmed, and yet we need to stay focused and alert and continue to think and function. This links back to the distinction I wrote about between self-in-relation-to-internal world vs -external world [44]. There might also be times when perceiving ourselves as a collection of multiple selves is more functional than as a unified whole self. Hence, even perceiving some parts of our experience as belonging to us and other parts being disowned, exiled, or belonging elsewhere.

At the end of the day, if we are starting from the assumption that our brain is in the business of keeping us alive, then why would it not evolve ways of more successfully achieving that? Remember from Chapter 1, 'It's better to be safe than sorry'. Coming back to our evolutionary scene that we described right at the beginning of the book, where there were a group of caveman ancestors sitting around relaxing by their cave. Which of these ancestors are more likely to have survived in this environment of looming and potential danger incoming at any time, and from any direction? The ones who always took time to calculate the precise cause-and-effect accuracy of the danger before they acted? Or the ones who sometimes used accuracy (when they had the luxury of time) and otherwise used guesses, hunches, and impulses?

A predictive processing account of voice-hearing and delusions

Let's return to the example mentioned previously in this chapter, where, after a run, my dog frantically rushes around the room barking and growling for 30 seconds. Perhaps her perception has created for her an imaginary threat (which to me looks like the rug, or a sock or a slipper). Although my perception is of a harmless piece of fabric or footwear, to my dog's perception this may be a threat object which provides her with a clear target and orientation with which to release her excess energy and complete her emotional process.

In *predictive processing* models, all perception is constructed. In other words, we might say all perception is hallucinated. We only have to go back and look at the visual illusions on page 14 to remind ourselves that our brain is making up its own perceptual reality. Sometimes it's pretty accurate (it's trying to reduce prediction error as much as possible), but at other times, there are evolutionary imperatives that override accuracy, particularly when fear is involved and survival is at stake. Seth suggests that the main task of our brain's perceptual system is to keep the internal conditions of the body as stable as possible in order to survive and satisfy basic biological needs. And from this premise, he argues that our perceptions can be thought of as either 'controlled' or 'controlling' hallucinations [47]. The 'controlled' bit implies that the hallucinations are tied to, and constrained by, reality (in that constant error-checking and updating happens) – so they are not totally free to run wild! The 'controlling' bit implies that the hallucinations can also activate responses in us and drive actions in a particular direction. Hence, sometimes perception is about best-guessing, and sometimes it's about controlling and regulating the body.

For me, this is why it's so important to consider the role of underlying (evolved) motivational states in driving perceptions and actions. If I am feeling fearful, and my body's evolved threat system is switched on, then my brain might create perceptions for me that drive protective action to bring my body back to a safe and stable state. Hence, in the *Compassion Focused Therapy* approach, which is rooted in a scientific understanding of evolved motives and mentalities, we pay particular attention to what motivation systems are online. Is the threat–protection system online? Is this a competitive system? Or a caring system? Whichever of these motivational systems are switched on will shape how perception and action is operating. In a recent journal article, we provided a synthesis of *Predictive Processing* and *Compassion Focused chairwork* for voice-hearing, which describes in more detail the intersection between motivation and perception [11].

Perceptions of hearing distressing voices ('auditory hallucinations'), and perceptions of the presence of threat ('paranoid delusions') could be understood as models to either *predict the causes of* threat signals in our body, or to *activate* threat emotions and actions. Or both. In line with all the other controlled explosion objectives we have identified in this book, these remote detonators could be used to support many functions: from *preparing and bracing* for threat, to *habituating, numbing, and dissociating*, to *catalysing and discharging* threat emotion. The remote detonation option may be a handy bit of kit to achieve these same functions, but just a bit more powerfully, for example, when more urgent or greater force is needed.

There might be times when our brain is detecting emotional signals from our body which are telling us that certain bodily needs are not being met, and therefore demand urgent action from us. Perceiving an 'externally' located threat (such as a voice located, say, to the right of my body) might be an effective way to produce the action required. The threat signal (the voice) increases certainty and control by providing a clear source, orientation, and action options. So here, the function of the voice-hearing perception is twofold. On the one hand, it is serving to *amplify* threat signals in our body (make them more precise); and on the other hand, it is providing a model that *orientates* and *mobilises* a direction for our actions.

Back to our cavemen around the fire ... Could it be that the ones who survived and passed on their genes are the ones who could rapidly self-stimulate their bodies into protective action via hallucinated threats?

Threat overlays on our perceptual map

In the next doodle, I was playing around with idea of having 'threat overlays' on our perceptual map. What I mean by this is considering our brain as having some specific threat templates (or prototypes) that it can apply as an overlay onto our perceptual reality when we are in significant danger. This overlay can instantly provide us with both a source of danger and a clear orientation and route to safety. This 'overlay' concept has really helped me personally think about the function of people's voice-hearing and delusion-believing experiences. What if we could think of voice-hearing and delusion-believing experiences as overlays: there is a threat source coupled with its own (predefined) action and response plan. When we are in danger, we can apply this perceptual overlay, and immediately our protective actions are set in motion. When I work clinically with people with psychosis, and when I am training other psychosis clinicians on this topic, I am always curious to draw attention towards the actions that are being activated in the voice-hearing or delusion-believing experience. I am asking the question: *"when you are hearing this voice, what feelings and responses are being activated in your body?"* And then the following question: *"do these feelings, sensations, and urges in your body remind you of any other experiences from your past?"*

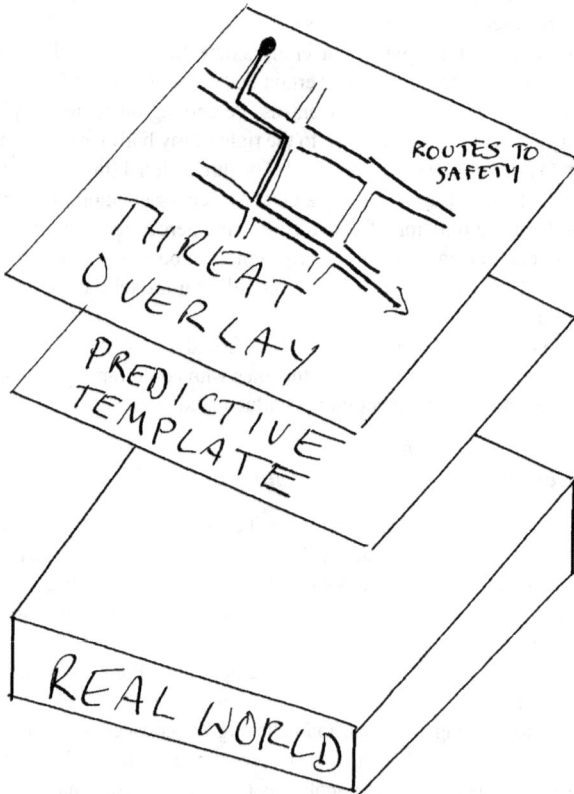

DOODLE: "Threat overlays on our perceptual map"

These kinds of questions, which pay particular attention to the body signals and body triggers, can really help the person to start making links to the memories, relationships, and relational traumas that might be behind these experiences. In terms of controlled explosions, the '**HARM AVERTED**' can often be connected back to the person's fears of re-traumatisation.

HARM CREATED: *I perceive the presence and sound of a voice criticising me*

HARM AVERTED: *Being vulnerable and unprepared for people's hostility and rejection*

Sometimes the 'threat overlays' could be there to help us deal with external threats (in the external world), and other times they could be to help us deal with internal threats (from our own emotions and body). So, for example, a threat overlay could shape our perception in such a way that helps us avoid awakening a buried feeling in our body. The danger being that if we accessed and activated that feeling, then it would set in motion a number of physical sensations and behavioural actions that could put us in danger. So here, the 'routes to safety' etched into this overlay would be more about creating suppression and dissociation.

What if we try to attack or banish our inner attackers?

If another person is attacking us or seeking to harm us, and there is no way to escape, then it is important for us to be able to defend ourselves. We might need to put up a firm boundary or barrier to prevent the harm, or we might need a strong push back to weaken or subdue the attacker. It might be a good idea to banish, expel (or even eliminate) the attacker to make sure they can no longer harm us in the future. But do these same principles apply to an internal attacker? What if the attacker is one part of us attacking another part of us? Would it still be a good idea to fight it? To attack the attacker? This is a question that my colleague Tobyn and I were contemplating in our *chairwork* article [11]. We described how different models of psychotherapy have developed quite different, often opposing, views on this issue. Many models would encourage taking a prohibitive stance, suggesting that these parts are not wanted, should not be there, and should either be ignored, suppressed, or expelled from our mind. Other models would encourage an inclusive stance, suggesting that these parts are there for a reason (perhaps protective), which we can seek to understand, work with, learn from, and integrate in a helpful way.

One of the problems here is that this debate has led various models to develop quite hard lines on this: for example, *we always* aim to weaken the attacker through assertiveness, confrontation, challenge, and push back; *we never* engage with an internal attacker; *we always* engage with these parts on the assumption that there must be a positive or helpful function; *under no circumstances* can these be viewed as helpful or protective. These kinds of rigid directives are actually quite restrictive and problematic, in my view, because in reality, it depends. There are so many contextual factors to consider when choosing the most helpful stance towards an inner attacker, and it would be far more beneficial to keep *a range of* options open. Indeed the wisest option to choose today might be very different to the wisest option to choose next month. Why limit the range with a hard-and-fast rule for how 'we should' engage with a perceptual experience, when every perceptual experience is unique, and occurs within a unique context of time, external (environmental) setting, and internal (bodily) state?

In our article [11], we presented a PP account of distressing voice-hearing, drawing attention to both roles in the voice-hearing relationship (a threat-giver and a threat-receiver). This helped us to highlight the potential importance of our body's threat signals in activating and maintaining the perception of hearing a voice. If it is the case that our own body signals of threat emotion and competitive action are the things driving a voice-hearing perception – the (hallucinated) perception of an attacker – then clearly taking a combative approach towards a voice would only risk amplifying these attacks. The more we try to overpower and silence a voice, the more our brain detects the signals of a conflict (from our body) and gives us the perceptions that predict or 'fit' this current threat. An alternative to this, which I have been investigating in the *Compassion Focused Therapy* approach to voice-hearing, is to focus on creating body signals of calmness, safeness and groundedness, and help people move away from competitive, conflictual relationships with voices, towards relationships that are more collaborative and co-operative. However, although moving from competitive to collaborative relationships may be a longer-term goal, it is important that at any one time, we still retain the *full range* of response options that are available to us. If, for example, we are being attacked relentlessly by a voice, then it might be helpful to start some disengagement or boundary-setting as a first step, even if it was just to allow ourselves some time to restore an experience of safeness and groundedness in the body in order to think about the best way to proceed. So rather than getting pulled into a power battle or conflict with the voice, we might respectfully initiate a pause or break, with the intention to resume the communication later. So, in this example, there is still an overarching intention to collaborate, but also a recognition that collaboration in this moment may not be possible or helpful due to the intensity of the body triggers and threat emotions.

It might be helpful here to compare this to a situation where a married couple are having an argument. Their emotions are high, their bodies are sending threat signals, their brains are predicting threat perceptions that are rapidly escalating the situation into more extreme positions of disagreement. The louder one person becomes, the bigger the response activated in the other, and the more amplified, exaggerated versions of these two 'roles' are being played out. This couple could keep amplifying the argument by staying right there in the heat of the conflict, getting louder and more extreme. Or they could terminate the argument altogether by walking away. However, neither of these options would really resolve anything. The chances are that this is an important conversation to have – there is a disagreement here that both parties feel strongly about. And if they are able to realise the importance of this – that this is a disagreement which needs to be identified, communicated, and discussed so they can find a way forward – then neither the 'escalating' option, nor the 'shutting down' option, would be helpful. Another option would be to take a 5-minute break – to walk away, but with the intention of returning to the conversation. For this couple, they know that just these 5 minutes of allowing their bodies to ground and settle will open the opportunity to effectively articulate and communicate the point they are trying to make, whilst also being able to hear the other person's point. So, the decision to disengage (to walk away) is not an attempt to avoid or suppress, but is a crucial step towards engagement and resolution.

Returning to the voice-hearing relationship, this is why being able to access our *full range* of responses and actions may be required to move the relationship in a more helpful direction. Sometimes creating distance, sometimes getting closer and leaning right in. Sometimes engaging with a firmer, more assertive voice tone, sometimes with a softer voice tone. This will change day-to-day, moment-to-moment. This diagram illustrates how, in the *Compassion-Focused Therapy* approach to voice-hearing, we would aim to recruit and train a compassionate part (a compassionate self or compassionate other) to take the role of a *third person* perspective. In this role, we would train compassionate qualities, such as wisdom, strength and courage, and use this wise, compassionate stance to understand the voice-hearing conflict, and to guide the relationship towards what is helpful and needed.

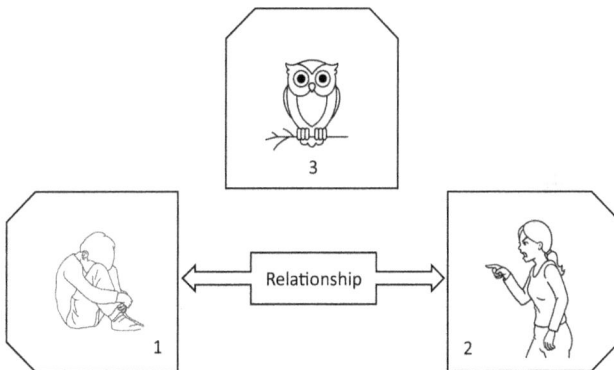

1. A profile of the body arousal and action urge that is switched on in the voice-hearing experience
2. A profile of the voice
3. A profile of the compassionate other

Three parts that could form the basis of a compassion-focused chairwork intervention [11]. Reproduced with permission

The role of compassion in approaching, understanding, and addressing controlled explosions will be a key focus of Chapter 6, where there will be plenty of suggestions and ideas, as well as worksheets and scripts, to help guide you through. As we have now concluded our tour of Bomb Squad HQ, we can remove our helmets, take a deep breath, and prepare our curiosity for what on earth we might do with these inner troublemakers.

Part III

A compassionate guide to defusing controlled explosions

Chapter 6

Approaching our inner controllers with compassion

Chapter summary

This chapter guides us through some ideas for what might be a more helpful approach to relating to our bomb squad and *controlled explosions*, which after all, are understandable (albeit problematic) aspects of this tricky evolved brain of ours. This chapter will draw partly on an approach informed by *Compassion Focused Therapy*, as well as other trauma-focused approaches, involving stages of (1) noticing, (2) understanding the function, and (3) helping. In the approach presented, the suggestion will be less about 'bombing the bomb squad', and more about bringing understanding and compassion to what's behind it or driving it – for example, moving towards identifying and addressing the 'bigger harm' or emotional pain that is being avoided or protected. The key idea is that the more we bring this into our compassionate focus and care, the less we might require controlled explosions to protect us.

Approaches we may be tempted with (and unintended consequences)

Bombing the bomb squad or struggling with the struggle

It may be quite tempting for us to enter into a struggle with the struggle. For example, we might feel ashamed about our procrastination, or we might feel drawn into a scrap or battle with our inner critic. We might try to hide or deny things that we are doing that cause harm to our bodies. This 'struggle with the struggle' can quickly descend into even greater problems for us. If we are ashamed about our procrastination, for instance, we might avoid even thinking about the thing we are procrastinating, which of course will lead to further procrastination. If we

DOI: 10.4324/9781003559924-10

start trying to silence our perfectionism, we could become even more worried that something terrible will happen. In Chapters 3 and 5, we considered some of the reasons why we must be cautious about taking a combative approach towards a self-critic or a voice, as this may risk amplifying our competitive emotions and threat signals, and lead to even stronger attacks. The same is true for most, if not all, the other *controlled explosions* in this book. The bottom line is that *controlled explosions* are rooted in the threat system. They are protective. They are there for a reason. If we simply charged in and forced the bomb squad away from their protective duties, we would be adding *more* conflict into the mix, not less. Adding more fuel to the threat fire. Removing one bomb squad member would likely lead to another one springing up in its place, because the underlying reasons for needing *controlled explosions* in the first place have not yet been addressed or resolved. Even worse, if we started treating the bomb squad as 'the enemy' and a threat to us, then we might set up a cascade of explosions, where new controlled explosions are needed to protect us from the old ones. This can quickly spiral into a self-destructive cycle that just keeps distancing us further and further away from the actual *root* of the problem – which is the reason why a 'bigger' harm needed protecting in the first place. Although tempting, bombing the bomb squad may not be the best approach, certainly not as a long-term solution to uprooting the harm and the causes of harm.

The bomb squad are not our enemies. They are protecting something big; something hurt; something wounded or painful. In many cases, it may be linked to a difficult life experience – a threat, a trauma, or a tragedy. An unmet need from childhood, perhaps, or some other emotional conflict that is still unresolved from earlier in our life. There is some part of our internal world that is still holding an unresolved and feared threat. It may be locked away in our body somewhere, and our brain has been working tirelessly to keep it safe. Desperately believing and hoping that everything will be ok as long as it can just keep building a world around this, where this wound is safe and out of harm's way. Scanning the world for threats, creating controlled explosions, sabotaging things in our life that could potentially put us at risk of being exposed to that (bigger) threat, hurt, or pain we are holding.

The controlled explosions do harm us though – we must not lose sight of that either. That I hope is very clear by now, from the numerous examples presented in this book, including some of the most serious and severe cases. So, while the bomb squad are not our enemies, we must be careful not to veer too far in the other direction either, of romanticising them. Yes, they do a protective job for us. But no, we certainly wouldn't want them to be our compassionate guides or life coaches, and we wouldn't choose them as caring teachers for our children. We don't want to fight them, but nor do we want to appease them and let them carry on controlling, dictating, and sabotaging our lives. There are choices we have here. There are middle options. There are ways of understanding and approaching our inner controllers that could lead to harm reduction, as well as to transformation and growth.

One of the central problems with the bomb squad and controlled explosions is that they are firmly rooted in the threat system. They come from a place of fear and protection. So, while they are incredibly important in serving a protective function for us, they are quite narrow-minded and blinkered in their approach. If the motto of the evolved brain is 'better safe than sorry', the motto of the bomb squad would be 'protect at all costs'. The bomb squad are exceptional at the job they have been deployed to do, but they are not able to see the bigger picture. They do not have the benefit of 'a view from the balcony' (see diagram). This is why we cannot rely on the bomb squad as being our best guides, coaches and teachers towards transformation and growth. So if we don't want to fight and banish them, and we definitely don't want them to be in charge of our lives either, what can we do with them?

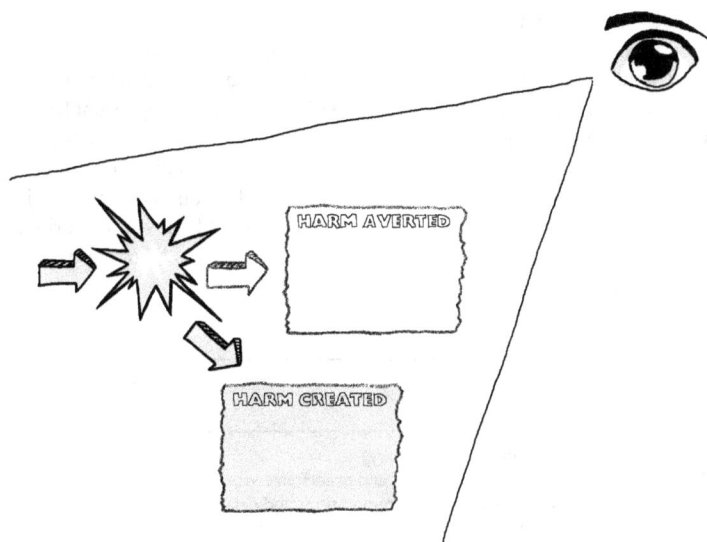

DOODLE: "A view from the balcony"

Identifying the protective function (and the 'bigger' threat)

First and foremost, we can work with the bomb squad to increase our awareness and understanding; awareness about the self-sabotaging, -criticising, and -harming behaviours that are happening in our lives, consciously or unconsciously; and understanding the functions they serve. That's what this book is about. It's not a self-help book. It is a self-awareness and self-understanding book. There is nothing in this book that tells you how you *should* self-help, or what self-help choices are right for you. As the author, I don't know what your versions of harm are, or your help needs. But becoming aware of your own controlled explosions is the start of you being able to determine your own self-help. Developing an understanding opens up choices for you. *"Do I accept this controlled explosion as a way of managing this 'bigger' threat?" "Do I want to address/resolve the underlying threat?" "Or do I want to switch to a different strategy for managing this?"* This book is not going to tell you which choice is best for you. Only you know that. And the best choices for you might change with time and circumstances. For example, if you are using a controlled explosion strategy that harms you physically, you might decide to accept that harm to continue for a period, while you build up the resources that are required to address the bigger fears, threats, and traumas that lie underneath. There is no right or wrong, but I hope this book provides you with some new insights and understandings to help you make wise and informed choices for yourself. In particular, the worksheets in Appendix 3 might help you to identify and map out your choices in a clearer and more systematic way.

In terms of awareness and understanding, it may be that you have already been building this up for yourself as you've been reading through the previous chapters. You may have been resonating with some of the many examples I've shared. However, I appreciate it's hard to keep everything in mind, so here is a table just to recap the full 15 areas we have covered. If you like, you can make a note of the ones that seemed to resonate the most for you as they were being introduced. Did you feel yourself particularly interested, moved, or intrigued by any of these? In what way did it resonate? And were there any specific examples of your own that jumped out at you?

	Does this resonate with me?
Derails my life and plans (self-sabotage)	
CERTAINTY-SEEKER – affirmed self and predictable world	
PROCRASTINATOR – distractions, temptations and delays	
PERFECTIONIST – exceptional standards and error-checks	
PESSIMIST – low expectations and anticipate problems	
CHAOS-CREATOR – drama, chaos and catastrophe	
Harms me psychologically (self-criticism)	
IMPROVER – a self-improvement response	
BLAMER – a feeling of agency and control	
DISCHARGER – a fight-or-flight response	
SUBMITTER – a submissive response	
DISSOCIATOR – a dissociative response	
Harms me physically (self-harm)	
MODIFIER – body modifications	
REORIENTATOR – diversions and reorientation	
PAIN-RELIEVER – natural pain relief and numbing	
HABITUATOR – desensitisation, habituation and mastery	
CATALYST – amplify, speed up and complete	

After the noticing and awareness step comes the understanding step. For this step, the method we have been using in this book is to map out the controlled explosion into its two key aspects: the **HARM CREATED**, and the **HARM AVERTED**. The harm created is generally a bit easier to map because that's the thing you have identified as your self-sabotaging, self-criticising, or self-harming pattern. Mapping the harm averted might be harder because it is not necessarily something you are aware of all the time, or even at all. It might be quite hidden. It might even be something you have been averting for years and have successfully buried under many layers of avoidance. So how can we identify this harm? This is where the bomb squad may be able to help.

Collaborating with the bomb squad

We want to understand more about the possible function of our controlled explosions, but rather than making random guesses in the dark, why not just ask the ones who know? We have recognised that there's likely to be some protective function (a feared harm that's being avoided), but we don't necessarily know what. However, the bomb squad certainly do. This is their purpose; their whole life's work; their *raison d'être*. They are highly (and exclusively) focused on this threat and possibly have been for many years. Perhaps the best chance we have of uncovering the roots and the function of *controlled explosions* is through engagement and collaboration with the bomb squad themselves. If we approach the bomb squad with conflict and fighting, or with ignoring, pushing away, and avoiding, then we may lose our best chance of discovering, unlocking, and uprooting what's underneath – what's really been driving our self-sabotaging, -criticising, and -harming actions all along.

The fact that you can't necessarily see the bigger threat underneath is because the bomb squad have been doing such an excellent job at protecting you from it. This is the main reason they were deployed in the first place. To keep it hidden and out of your awareness. But bomb squads do not need to be *permanently* deployed on the same job. The role of a bomb squad member may only be needed for a period – more like a temporary position. For example, it might have been highly functional to protect you from a feared threat while you were going through a difficult stage of your life. Maybe during a period at school, or in the context of a tricky relationship, or a job, or a transition. Maybe 30 or 40 years have passed since then. The reason why the bomb squad member is still around today is not because they take pleasure in continually harming you, it's because you haven't yet resolved the underlying trauma or threat. It's still very much alive in your mind and body somewhere. When you find and process this threat, it can be resolved. And it's only then that the bomb squad will feel safe enough that their work is done, and that their *controlled explosions* are no longer required.

One of the choices we have, therefore, is to work with the bomb squad, to collaborate with them, to get a clearer understanding of what are these threats and fears, and to get an understanding of our needs. What is needed to start feeling safe in that area of my life? When safeness is felt in that area, and the threat system starts to settle, the bomb squad will naturally settle too. The 'threat' fuel that has been driving our body, perceptions, and actions for so long will start to become blended and balanced with a fresh stream of 'safeness'. It is when the bomb squad feel *safeness* that they'll know it's time to defuse their controlled explosions, open up the hatches of their containment vessels, file away their threat overlays, and bring their remote detonators back to base.

Remember, the bomb squad don't have the benefit of the 'view from the balcony'. They cannot look at the situation from this broader vantage point. Nor are they motivational states, so cannot change in their attitudes and intentions. The bomb squad are linked to brain states, threat emotions, and protective (defensive) actions, so will just keep protecting and protecting until we can show them (and allow them to feel for themselves) that there is nothing more to protect. This is why the process of collaboration and co-operation can be a useful route. Collaboration is about bringing different parties together who can offer different expertise to the discussion. The bomb squad are experts in protection. They know your biggest fears. They hold extensive records about your traumas, wounding memories, and all the threats that must be averted at all costs. What you bring to the table is a different wisdom and expertise. You know about your goals, your plans, ambitions, and the things that are important to you in life. You also have an understanding about the passage of time, and about the concept of how something that may be terrifying for a young child, might not be so terrifying for a grown-up adult. You have the benefit of seeing the different contexts of past, present, and future. Bringing these 'wisdoms' together – yours and the bomb squad's – could make for a very strong team. But what could make it *even* stronger is a 'third party' helper too – a compassionate guide who can oversee, mediate, and support the collaboration.

A compassionate 'third party' view from the balcony

We said before that the bomb squad are restricted by not having access to the 'view from the balcony'. The importance of the balcony view cannot be understated, because it's from this vantage point that we can see context. We can see pros and cons of certain actions. For example, where something may have advantages in the short term, but disadvantages in the long term. And how it may be that long-term costs might far outweigh the short-term benefits. We can understand that every decision involves trade-offs, we can consider different aspects and angles, and it's from this perspective that we can make wise choices.

We can certainly appreciate the importance of having a view from the balcony. But is that enough? In the *Compassionate Focused Therapy* approach, we would go one step further and really focus on what *kind* of view – what is the orientation and nature of this view from the balcony? What is the stance and the intention behind it? What is the motivational texture we are bringing from this vantage point? Maybe simply being on the balcony is not enough, because, in theory, we could go the balcony and develop quite a critical attitude or stance towards what we are looking at. Do we really want a critical stance when we are trying to build a collaborative relationship with a part of us that holds information about our personal traumas? How would that turn out? Therefore, we want to make sure that this balcony view is being used to guide the collaborative process and move it forwards in a helpful direction. This is a caring intention. A motivation to collaborate, co-operate, and to care.

To instil these compassionate motivations into a process like this is not just 'a given'. It takes time, effort, and intentionality. Remember from the first chapter, our brain has a natural habit of tricking us and biasing our perceptions of reality. If left to its own devices, it would naturally veer towards 'better safe than sorry' biases, especially in the presence of threat emotions (which of course there will be in this collaboration – that's the central topic!). So, it is probably not wise to just leave it to chance that our brain will naturally take a caring and co-operative stance when faced with our biggest fears and traumas. However, we can train it. We can do what we can to give our brains the best chance of accessing a compassion standpoint. We can use all our best understandings from years of scientific research, as well as years of human experience and ancient wisdom, to create the optimum conditions for compassion. This is where so much credit and gratitude are owed to the master of this area, Paul Gilbert; the person who has read almost every book and scientific paper there is to read on how to create the bio-psycho-social conditions for a compassionate mind. These studies, learnings, and wisdoms are what have been compiled by Paul, for all our benefit, into the processes and practices of *Compassion Focused Therapy* [48–50].

In the *Compassion Focused Therapy* approach, the model offered in our Balanced Minds therapy centre, we train and practise cultivation of a compassionate mindset, which we operationalise as either a 'compassionate self' or 'compassionate other'. There are various body-based, psychological, and behaviour exercises that are involved to support this process, referred to collectively as *Compassionate Mind Training* [51–53]. We will equip the compassionate self with the kinds of qualities that are necessary for engaging with distress and suffering, with a commitment to help. Hence, when thinking about the remit for the kind of character we would want on our balcony, we needn't look much further than the compassionate self. As shown in the doodle, the compassionate self can help *create the conditions* for a collaborative process of discovery.

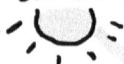

VIEW FROM THE BALCONY

COMPASSIONATE
SELF oR OTHER

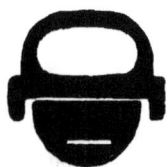
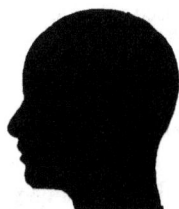

Creating the conditions for a
collaborative process of discovery.
With the aim of
understanding the
protective function
of controlled explosions
and the 'bigger' threat
that's driving them.

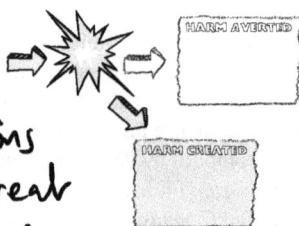

DOODLE: "The compassionate 'third party' view from the balcony"

In Appendix 4, there is a series of seven imagery exercise scripts that you can use to create your own visual scenes and interactions that relate to key topics and processes in this chapter. The inclusion of these scripts provides an option for those readers among you who wish to try engaging more experientially with the ideas presented. (These exercises are also available to access as audios uploaded on my author website, www.charlieheriotmaitland. com). However, doing these experiential exercises is not an essential part of reading this book. You won't lose anything if you choose not to try out these practices, so it's entirely up to you. You might prefer to just read them through out of interest, rather than engaging with any imagery practice per se. The first four scripts guide you in creating the conditions for compassion, specifically creating a compassionate self and then preparing three scenes in which your compassionate self may be able to help: a *view from the balcony*; a *room with chairs*; and a *calm place*. The other three scripts guide you in using your compassionate self to meet a bomb squad member who is creating a controlled explosion in your life, along with three of your different 'selves' who may have useful insights to deepen your understanding of this controlled explosion and how to help: your *day-to-day self*; your *younger self*; and your *future* self.

Engaging with a member of the bomb squad

First, we can spend a bit of time profiling the character we are interested in engaging with. You can refer back to page 124 where we listed them all in a table, and you thought about which ones were resonating for you. We have already got some names for these characters, so you can stick with these names if you like, or if you'd rather make up your own names that's fine too. You can then use your imagination to come up with a few other ideas for what this character would be like. In this book, I have depicted them all as wearing helmets, but that's just how my imagination works! For you, it might be different. Would your character have a helmet, or would you change that to something else? What about their facial expression? What do you imagine would be the voice tone of this character? What about gender? Age? Any other physical characteristics that you notice? Do you imagine them sitting down or standing? Where are they? What's the setting? What kind of body language do they have?

The reason we are spending some time profiling this bomb squad member is that this will create more options for you in the various methods you can use for engaging with them. For example, some people prefer using imagery methods to set up an encounter with a different part of them. Others might prefer a letter-writing exchange, where you communicate between parts of yourself with written messages. Voice messages back and forth would be another option. Some might prefer drama and acting techniques, where you could 'play the role' of the character, acting and talking out loud, and then switch over to a different role (maybe moving to a different chair) and then respond as the other character. These kinds of role-play, drama, and so-called 'chairwork' techniques can really help to bring your body experience and physical sensations into play, which as we've seen throughout this book, have such a key role in self-defeating perceptions and actions.

Your compassionate self, which has its own profile too (imagery, facial expression, body posture, and so on) can be used in multiple ways to support this engagement with the bomb squad character. It can stay on the 'balcony', and take more of a reflective role, maybe offering some general guidance and support for the communication between you and the bomb squad member. Or the compassionate self can get more involved if you like and can be used as a role from which to engage or communicate directly with the characters in the scene. For example, this could be asking questions directly to the bomb squad member about its function, and what it's trying to keep you safe from. Or this could be asking questions directly to you about what that feels like, being harmed and sabotaged in your life. You could practise switching roles as both the giver and receiver of compassion. The more the compassionate self is practised and is more able to influence these exchanges with its calm authority, wisdom, and caring attitude, the more 'safeness' feelings are gradually flowing in and around the system. Our body can start detecting that 'safeness' signals are possible, even in these most difficult 'conflict' zones that were historically reserved for threat.

Appendix 4.5 provides a script for setting up a compassionate encounter with your bomb squad member. In terms of discovering the function of controlled explosions, the kinds of questions we might be interested in asking this character are as follows:

- *How long have you been in my life?*
- *Do you remember when you first showed up in my life?*
- *Why then? What was going on for me at that time?*
- *What are your main concerns about me, my life, my future?*
- *What are your greatest fears?*
- *What is the most important thing about the job you do for me?*
- *If you couldn't do your job for me one day (for example, if you went away on vacation), what would be your greatest fear about what might happen?*
- *If I didn't have you around protecting me anymore, what would be the fear?*
- *If we could press pause in the exact millisecond right before you create a controlled explosion, what would be the emotion and sensation in my body?*
- *What words would you use to describe that feeling?*
- *Where is that located in my body? Can you point to that now?*
- *Does that feeling remind you of anything else in my life? For example, is there any time in my childhood when I had a similar feeling?*

You could try using any of the techniques mentioned above (imagery, letter-writing, role-play) to set the scene for having this communication, or, to start with, you could just simply try writing some answers to these questions directly, as if you're completing a questionnaire. But remember you are attempting to generate your answers from the perspective of your inner protector – the bomb squad member, so trying to put yourself in their shoes and (threat) mindset as best as you can. And remember that your compassionate self is always there on hand and ready to help, and to step in whenever is needed. So, for example, if anything starts to feel too overwhelming or difficult, you can come back to the role of the compassionate self and reconnect with your calm breathing rhythm and your grounded body posture. If you notice that you are getting frustrated and angry with your bomb squad character, and you feel this is escalating into a conflict or fight, this might be a good moment to just stabilise your breathing and posture, and to get grounded again. This is not about trying to suppress the angry feeling – definitely not – because the angry feeling is likely to be an important and necessary thing to feel, and for a good reason. But this is a moment where, with the support of your compassionate self, you can *be with* that angry feeling and identify where in your life some of this anger might be rooted or coming from. Noticing it, allowing it to be there in your body. If you just 'discharged' the anger towards the squad member, then not only may you escalate the conflict, but you may also miss a prime opportunity to connect with the anger and identify its *true* context and source.

Once you've identified the 'bigger threat' – the underlying harm that's being averted – you will be able to complete your own version of the controlled explosions template. As you will recall, the two main elements are:

HARM CREATED: ....

HARM AVERTED: ....

Compassion for the deeper harms, and the threatened or unmet needs

The underlying harms (averted) are the things that have been driving your controlled explosions. Without you even knowing it, your brain has been carefully constructing your life around the imperative to avert these deeper harms – to avoid re-experiencing these harmed or wounded parts of you. Your perceptual structures, your behaviour, and your self-sabotaging patterns, have all been shaped and textured around the goal of protecting these. Often the reason why these parts were hurt so profoundly in the first place, earlier in your life, is because they were linked to some of your core needs – things that you have always needed, wanted, yearned, and longed for. These are the things that can hurt us the most; for example, things like our need to be loved and cared for, or our need for belonging and acceptance. So, our biggest harms are often connected to experiences where our core needs were threatened or unmet. And it's these underlying threats, harms, and needs that require our compassion and care.

You can use the same techniques as before – imagery, writing, or role play – to create a scene to explore these connections between harms and needs, again with the help of your compassionate self. The scene we developed previously was set for an encounter with your bomb squad member (with the aim of learning about its fears, functions, and the underlying harms it has been protecting). This time, the scene could be set for an encounter with your younger self who is feeling vulnerable or hurt. The aim here could be to learn about how these underlying harms may be connected to core needs of yours that were threatened or unmet. Again, your compassionate self can provide a caring container for this, and help you approach and texture this exploration with care motivations and qualities such as strength and wisdom. In Appendix 4.6, there is a suggested imagery exercise script I've developed for meeting your younger self if you would like to try this out. The following extract from the script demonstrates how this exercise aims to direct your focus towards unmet needs:

> *As the compassionate self, you want to help, and you want to understand more about these harms experienced by your younger self, and why it was so important for these to be protected ... You want to understand how these underlying harms and fears may be linked to core needs of yours that were threatened or not met.*

(Appendix 4.6)

Here are some sample questions that you could ask your younger self to help you link your deeper harms and fears to some of your basic younger needs:

- *What memories are linked to that scary or uncomfortable feeling in your body?*
- *When did you first feel that?*
- *Why was that so painful and hurtful for you at the time?*
- *What was the need that you were longing for?*
- *What was the need that was threatened?*
- *What is the need that you wanted, but was not available, or taken away?*

Resolution through creating safeness and grieving loss

Resolving underlying harm can often involve two aspects: (i) creating safeness around the feared situation and feeling, and (ii) grieving the loss of having a core need in that situation that was unmet, denied, or dismissed. The first part, creating safeness, can send the signal to your brain and body that you no longer require the protective structures that were built (externally and internally) to avoid that fear. The second part, grieving, can allow you to let go of these same structures that you had been relying on to keep alive the hope that this need would one day be met.

In addition, there may be a third important process of resolving anger too, for example, anger towards the people who denied or dismissed your needs or were unable to meet them.

Here is a (simplified) illustration of how creating safeness might help us to shift our motivational and perceptual orientation away from a threat-focus to a safeness-focus:

Orientated around threat:	*"I fear being in a situation again where I might re-experience the painful feeling of a core need being unmet, denied, or dismissed"*
Orientated around safeness:	*"It'll be ok. I'm safe. I know that situation was hard, and I understand why it was so painful for me, but I'm going to be ok"*

And here is a brief illustration of how the grieving process might help us to move away from an orientation to a (thwarted) past need that we haven't been able to let go of yet, towards an orientation to a present and future need that we can build towards:

Orientated to denying and protecting a thwarted past need:	*"How can I avoid the feeling of a core need being unmet, denied, or dismissed?"*
Orientated to embracing and building a present and future need:	*"How can I gain the feeling of a core need being met, embraced, and supported?"*

The compassionate self can support us in the process of addressing and resolving the threats, fears, and needs from the past. Once these unmet needs are identified and resolved, it may be that the bomb squad's self-sabotaging, -criticising, and -harming patterns can naturally dissolve away. The resolution processes in relation to our younger self may take a number of forms. For example, it might require:

i Creating safeness for the fears and anxieties of the younger self
ii Grieving the sadness and losses of the younger self
iii Processing the anger and rage of the younger self.

The imagery script in Appendix 4.6, which sets up a compassionate encounter with our younger self, could lay a path to help you approach these needs and resolutions in a safe way.

Controlled explosions for transformation and growth

When it comes to *controlled explosions*, one of the main struggles we have is that we are operating in a biological and psychological landscape that has been specifically built around a threat. The whole structure of our brain, or at least the circuits within our brain, were constructed, shaped, and wired with the purpose of avoiding that fear. The controlled explosions have essentially been operating to keep that same structure intact. The phrase we used previously as a motto for the bomb squad was "protect at all costs". But protect what? Up until this point, we have just been referring to a general role of protecting *us* (i.e. me or you). But it might be helpful to dig a bit deeper into what exactly is being protected. Yes, it is *us*. You or me. But specifically, it's the 'old' version of us. The version that was hurt and afraid in the past. The bomb squad has been protecting a version of our brain organisation and neurocircuitry that is old and out-of-date.

It's a bit like a dedicated team of construction workers who have worked tirelessly to keep maintaining a wobbly old bridge that was built at the turn of the 1900s to accommodate horse and cart. However much maintenance this team has been doing to this bridge, week after week, year after year, it's still never really going to be equipped to deal with the 100,000 cars and lorries per day that are now needing to use the bridge in 2025. It is not for lack of hard work or maintenance effort and skill, but there's something fundamental about the basic infrastructure or design that is no longer adequate for the present day. You could send in hundreds of the finest maintenance workers in the world, but it's not going to change that fact. It's no-one's fault, but the clear and unavoidable truth is that we simply have to take down the old bridge and build a new one.

So now the day comes that you must go and share this news with the maintenance team. As you go along and knock on the door of their workstation, you are full of trepidation because you know that this will be a very sad and painful piece of news to deliver. You have to inform them that the decision has been made to destroy the bridge. This is going to be heart-wrenchingly sad for them. All those years of checking, fixing, painting, fortifying, protecting. All gone. Not only are they losing their beloved bridge, but they're losing all the many thousands of collective hours that they've spent protecting it and keeping it intact. It's a double loss. A triple loss would be if there are members of that team who had been secretly longing and dreaming that if they just kept maintaining the bridge for long enough, that one day – maybe, just maybe – the world might bring back travel by horse and cart.

These are the equivalent losses to those of us humans who are trying to overcome self-sabotage, self-criticism, and self-harm – for those of us who are trying to heal ourselves towards transformation and growth after something traumatic and painful. As with the maintenance team, we are having to let go of: (i) the old structures that have served us and kept us safe for so many years, (ii) the countless number of days, months, years we have lost keeping these structures intact through sabotaging, criticising, and harming ourselves, and (iii) the hopes, dreams, and fantasies that if we kept these structures intact for long enough, then our core needs for love, safeness, and connection would eventually be met. This is a big deal. We are talking about a triple loss. And yet, this may still be a wise route forward for us.

As I have said repeatedly in this book, however, there is no right or wrong choice here. And there is no way for me or anyone else to know what choice is right for you. This book is aiming to help improve your understanding of these things so that you can see more clearly into the causes of harm and suffering, and to help lay out for you some of the choices you have. These are your choices though, and only yours. But remember, if you're struggling with these choices, it can be so helpful to talk it through with someone, maybe a trusted friend, a family member, or a therapist. Maybe with your compassionate self too. These are not easy choices, and should not be rushed. Give it time.

Clearing the way for a new structure

The controlled explosions we have been exploring in this book are ones that seek to avoid a feared harm and therefore maintain an old structure that was built around the 'harm-avoidance' design. However, when the point arrives in our life that we are ready for a new structure – when we realise that harm-avoidance is no longer the design we want – we must remove the old structure to clear the way for a new one.

So how do we remove old bridges? Well of course with … *controlled explosions*! But these are controlled explosions of a slightly different nature in terms of their function. The underlying functions behind these controlled explosions are not solely to protect, but to make way for a new beginning. The focus is not on the past, but on the future. Referring back to the 'needs' table on page 133, the orientation is not towards denying or protecting the painful feeling of a past thwarted need, but towards embracing the needs of now and of the future.

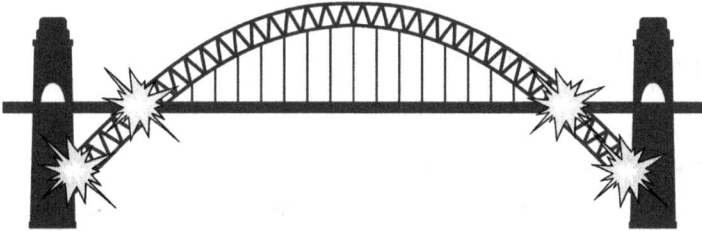

Using controlled explosions to enable a new structure to be built

Here we are invited to contemplate how controlled explosions can be used for transformation and growth. When the evolved threat system is no longer running the show, our attention can switch towards building, growing, and moving forward. There is still of course the loss, grieving, letting go, which is painful, and so again we can map this out in a similar two-part template to give us clarity about the inherent trade-off in this process:

HARM CREATED: *Breaking an old structure, with the loss and grief of letting go*

GROWTH OPENED: *Building a new structure better suited for the future*

In the earlier chapters, I have used some examples from my own personal bomb squad to help illustrate the kinds of threat-focused controlled explosions that we use, i.e. those that come with the objective of averting harm. Now that we have arrived at considering controlled explosions for transformation and growth, I am not going to go too far into my personal examples but would certainly like to share some of the thought processes that I might follow when I am looking into this for myself. What would I be looking for in my life? Maybe it would be times where I've had to replace an old, out-of-date, version of myself (a younger Charlie) with a new version that is more knowledgeable, strong, anchored, and better equipped to deal with the world as it is *now*. Maybe a pattern of behaviour that I used to use a lot in the past, but then later realised was based around an old fear and was no longer needed. For example, maybe a younger version who used to strive for achievements to get approval from others.

Then later, when realising this was no longer needed, building a newer version who could be loved without anything to do with their achievements. Maybe a younger version who used to avoid expressing their preferences or opinions due to a fear of being disliked. Then later, when realising this was based upon past threats or traumas, building a newer version who can feel safe to share more of themselves and their preferences. Maybe a younger version who used to hide and avoid, replaced by a newer version who can now show up and engage. A younger version who suppressed their needs, into a newer version who can not only understand their needs but also communicate and advocate for them.

Where do you get to when you follow this thought process for yourself? Is there a version of you – maybe a younger version – who was entirely built and structured around an old fear? Who is the past version that you can let go? Who is the new version that you can build?

From structures to circuits

In this diagram, there is visual comparison between (a) controlled explosions that maintain an existing circuit, and (b) controlled explosions that break down the old circuit and open the possibility for a new circuit.

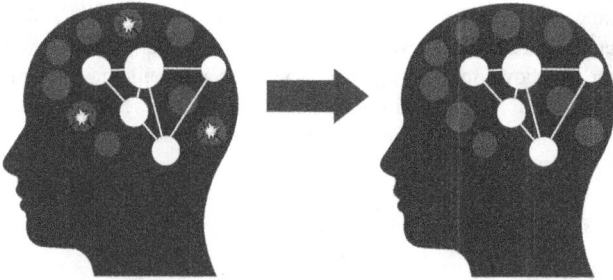

a) Controlled explosions that maintain an existing circuit

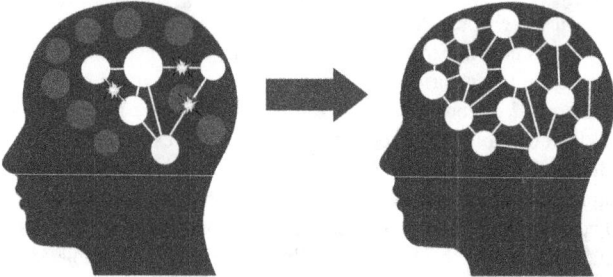

b) Controlled explosions that break down the old circuit and open the possibility for a new circuit

Controlled explosions for different functions

In the first image, (a), the brain's threat system is switched on, so the individual's sensory, perceptual, and cognitive worlds are fixed in a kind of fear-based 'holding pattern'. The controlled explosions in (a) are depicted as targeting areas around the circuits, so for example, pushing away other parts of us, such as emotional parts or needs, which might risk the integrity of the main threat circuit. In the second image, (b), the controlled explosions are shown to break the current 'closed' circuit down so that it loosens its grip on us and opens our brain up for new connections in the formation of a new circuit.

In (a), the bomb squad are of course dutifully threat focused. Along with their usual motto of *"protect at all costs"*, they may as well add in a *"circuit maintenance in progress"* banner along with a *"no entry"* sign. For the threat-focused bomb squad, re-traumatisation must never occur again, and anything that could present even the slightest risk of this happening must not be allowed near the circuit of awareness. For us, what this could mean is:

- **NO ENTRY** to certain needs, particularly those which could create a risk of me feeling the pain of those needs being thwarted
- **NO ENTRY** to certain emotions, particularly those which could create a risk of me behaving in a way that attracts harm or makes me a target
- **NO ENTRY** to certain hopes or ambitions, particularly those which could create a risk of me putting or finding myself in situations similar to the ones that hurt me.

So, in (a), the brain has essentially switched into a mode of trying to regulate how much emotion and pain can be allowed to enter the person's awareness. In our earlier accounts of *predictive processing* models (Chapter 1, which we then revisited in Chapters 3 and 5), we described how our brain's perceptual system is continually constructing models of reality for us. Sometimes these models are to 'fit' the world and reduce prediction errors, and other times they are to drive responses and actions that will keep the conditions of our body as stable as possible, ultimately for our survival and biological needs (what Anil Seth calls 'controlled' or 'controlling' hallucinations [10]). So, when we say that our brain is locked in a fear-based holding pattern, in which there is '**NO ENTRY**' for certain elements, from a *predictive processing* angle, these parts would be (literally) non-existent in our awareness. These elements would not be part of the constructed model of perception that the brain has selected for this moment. It's not that we are trying to ignore these parts or somehow deny or pretend they're not there. They are *literally* not there in the perceptual system.

Given that perception has a limited range, how then can we make the transition from (a) to (b)? From (a), maintaining the old circuits, to (b), building the new ones? How can we help our perceptual system to integrate other parts and elements that it cannot see, and as far as it's concerned, do not even exist?

For this to happen, there would firstly need to be a 'loosening the grip' (of control), a 'breaking down', and a 'letting go' of the existing circuit. And secondly, an 'opening up', 'making connections', and 'consolidating' of the new circuits.

i Loosening the grip, breaking down, and letting go

For loosening the grip of control, we would first need to establish safeness. It is our threat emotions that drive our need for control. The more threat there is, the more our grip tightens. So, introducing safeness and 'soothing system' emotions to regulate and balance the threat system would lay the foundations as an important first step. Understanding the neurophysiological patterns and processes of safeness, and how to access and cultivate these for ourselves, has been a central pillar in models such as *Polyvagal Theory* and *Compassion Focused Therapy*. Some of the key physiological processes identified as being linked to the 'safeness' experience include the ventral vagus nerve and heart rate variability. (If you are interested in diving deeper into this literature, on the *Polyvagal* side, some of the key research and work has been published by Steve Porges [54, 55] and Deb Dana [56]; and on the *Compassion* side, some of the key research and work has been published by Nicola Petrocchi, Marcela Matos, James Kirby, and colleagues [57–61].

For breaking down and letting go we would need courage. The breaking down of a safe, familiar, and well-rehearsed pattern is a bold step. We are likely to feel, at best, disorientated, and at worst, fractured and broken. We are willingly moving ourselves closer to out-of-control feelings, towards vulnerability and loss. This is hard. It takes our minds right back to the start of Chapter 2, where we met our first bomb squad member, the **CERTAINTY-SEEKER**. There will understandably be stress, tension, chaos, and uncomfortable feelings involved in breaking down our 'certainty' structures – these have been our anchors and our safety net. However, if we can bring wisdom and intentionality to this process, it need not be scary or overwhelming. If we are entering into 'breakdown' with a clarity of understanding and determination for why we are doing this, and with a caring motivation, this could be an enlivening experience and profoundly positive. This is very different to spiralling towards breakdown unwillingly and fearfully. Instead, we can remain connected to our intention that what we want here is something better for ourselves. We will return to this in the later section called "*Learning safe ways to let go of control*", where we will also come back to the idea of post-traumatic growth.

HARM CREATED: *Temporary pain and discomfort*

GROWTH OPENED: *Long-term adjustment and adaptation to the world*

There are also parallels here to a topic we were contemplating earlier with the **CHAOS-CREATOR** around the idea of 'creating chaos to rediscover order'. Remember we used a quote from *Star Wars*: *"One must destroy in order to create"* (page 50), which is very fitting for this current topic too. The crucial detail to note here is in the *intention*. The intention to create. To build. To transform. To grow. This is a caring intention, even if one segment of the route to this goal is destructive. Just like the destructive element of blowing up the old bridge to make way for a new one. There is a longer-term vision. If we only looked at these things with a very narrow and short-term focus we would see 'self-destruct'. However, as soon as we zoomed out and looked at the bigger vision, and a longer-term time frame, we would see 'self-care'. So, if we are taking the bold steps towards 'breaking down' and 'letting go', it is important to stay connected with our wise (and longer-term) intention for self-compassion and care.

ii Opening up, making connections, and consolidating

Building the new circuits will require an 'opening up' of new parts of our experience. New pockets and clusters of sensory–emotional information, in different parts of the brain, which will need to be activated simultaneously for connections to be made between them. This includes sensory signals that relate to the environment (external world) as well as sensory–emotional signals that relate to our body (internal world). This means allowing our mind to catch glimpses of new things externally and internally, things that may have been entirely absent from our perceptual models with the old circuit. In the external world, this might be a glimpse of seeing someone's care and kindness towards us. In the internal world, this might be a glimpse of having a desire, a feeling, or a need.

These glimpses might be the small building blocks with which we can start updating our perceptual models and creating new circuits in our brain. The process of *integration* of different parts, particularly the trickier (and riskier) parts that did not 'fit' in the previous model, will require compassion and care. For example, the parts that had previously been exiled will need to be welcomed back into our awareness, one-by-one. This could be a slow and steady procedure, depending on the degree of dissociation that was needed in the first place when the splitting and exiling of these parts took place. The compassionate self will be acting as a secure base and safe haven for this process of integration. As the unresolved parts move towards resolution, and the dissociated parts move towards integration, this will allow for new patterns, circuits, and structures to form. In terms of perceptual systems, as new interoceptive models (self in relation to internal world) are formed, this will allow the formation of new exteroceptive models (self in relation to external world).

Doing this work involves both the body and the world. We can be allowing ourselves to 'open up' to new feelings and start processing unresolved emotions, and at the same time, catching glimpses of new information in our environment and relationships. Both these layers contain some of the 'NO ENTRY' items that our previous perceptual models did not allow us to see. The process of opening to new feelings is particularly difficult, but several therapy models have developed innovative and creative techniques for doing this in a way that makes the process less overwhelming for people. In Eye Movement Desensitisation and Reprocessing (EMDR), for example, the therapist uses 'dual attention' techniques, such as hand movements or tapping techniques to ground a person in the here and now, while their brain is given the 'free reign' to make associative links with different memories, images, perceptual and conceptual information. By simultaneously activating different signals in different parts of the brain, new connections, networks, and circuits can begin to form. In EMDR therapy sessions, the therapist encourages their client to "go with that", as in just allow the brain to show you where it needs to go and what connections it needs to link up.

Using *Predictive Processing* terminology, we could speculate that perhaps these EMDR techniques are synchronising external (exteroceptive) and internal (interoceptive) models: An external perception (i.e. the therapist's hand-waving movement or tapping motion) is synchronised with an internal perception (i.e. the client's eye movement or tapping sensation). Having a synchronisation of the internal and external worlds would be a crucial part of rebuilding new circuits, as I argued in a 2011 article "Multi-level Models of Information Processing" [44]. EMDR is a technique I have trained in and occasionally use in my own therapy practice; however, for me, this would typically be used within the context of Compassion Focused Therapy – meaning that I would be seeking to bring the compassionate mind online first before using these processing techniques. For the reasons I described, I believe it's beneficial to orientate to the compassionate motivation first, to help facilitate any 'breaking down' or 'opening up' work. This principle applies equally to therapy as it does to self-help. In other words, if we initiate our self-help behaviour from a genuine motivation for self-compassion, this is more likely to be beneficial than if coming from a different motivation, say, for competitively gaining something, or for fearfully appeasing someone.

It is interesting to also consider here the processes that naturally occur in our brain when we sleep, particularly when we are dreaming in REM sleep (Rapid Eye Movement). The sleep researcher Matthew Walker suggests that REM sleep is a form of "overnight therapy" in that it's where our emotional memories can be safely activated and processed by our brain. In his book, *Why We Sleep* [62], Walker suggests that the brain creates a neurochemically calm environment (with reduced noradrenaline levels, for example) for our emotional processing to take place. He also describes how our dreaming in REM sleep can facilitate the abstract linking of information in different clusters of memories in other parts of our brain. This is similar to the process described earlier, where there is an opening up to new information. New associations and creative links can be formed between different clusters that don't necessarily exist in the same predictive templates. REM sleep may be a helpful setting for these new circuits to spontaneously start forming; a natural state where our brains can link up emotional themes and meanings, without being constrained by the usual limits and biases of perceptual experience while we're awake.

Future vision for a new structure

I have described the process of opening our brains up to information that was previously hidden from view. This can be either opening snippets of information from our past that our brains did not allow us to perceive or opening our potential to perceiving new information in the future. Once new information is unlocked and is available to us, new connections can start to be made. These new connections will then allow for new circuits to start forming – a process that will be happening naturally and spontaneously (perhaps even more so while dreaming in REM sleep, in our neurochemically curated incubator). In many ways, natural and spontaneous could be the ideal scenario for us here. As we have seen throughout this book, so much of our emotional suffering can come from our brain's attempts to control, and so allowing more spontaneity into this process might be a welcome and refreshing change. However, another important lesson we have learnt in the book is to not underestimate our brain's natural biases. Our brain, when left to its own devices, has quite a distorted relationship with both threat and reality (specifically, a natural attraction towards threat and a natural ambivalence towards reality). So, while it is important to allow some spontaneity and letting go of control, some light-touch facilitation in the desired direction of travel wouldn't go amiss. For example, perhaps there can be some future vision – even if it's just a vague gist – of what we want the new structure to look like.

When it comes to forming new brain circuits and building a new life, there is a bit of 'finding out' what our brain will do with new information and connections, combined with a little bit of light-touch guidance of what we *want* our brain to do with these. What circuits do we want to form? What experiences do we want to lay down now to influence our future perceptions and actions? What is the future version of ourselves and our life that we are moving towards?

Again, imagery is a powerful tool, and here it can be used as a nice way of combining a bit of natural spontaneity with a bit of guided intentionally. There is an imagery script in Appendix 4.7 that guides you through an exercise where you can meet your future self. Your future self is the version of you that you imagine has built a good structure for themselves. They are wise. They have opened up their brains to new information, which has helped them to learn more about the world and about themselves. They have made the new discoveries and have found the life structure, including the habits and routines, that work for them. If you are interested in trying this imagery exercise out for yourself, you will be guided through the experience of firstly seeing your future self in their daily life and then sitting down to have a conversation with them about some of the things they have learned. You may find out a bit about their interests, their daily routines, and how they live their life. You may also hear about some of the sacrifices they have had to make in building their new structure. These are the things they have had to let go of – the old structures, the old brain circuits and behaviour patterns that were no longer serving them.

Here is a list of some questions you might be interested in asking your future self:

- *What is your life like?*
- *What do you do each day?*
- *What did you have to let go of to get to where you are now?*
- *What sacrifices did you have to make?*
- *What advice would you give to the younger version of you?*
- *Which bits of your old life were requiring you to be someone you're not?*
- *What new structures and routines did you build?*
- *What advice would you give to start following the path into the life you've created?*
- *Is there anything else you have learnt?*
- *Is there anything else you want to share with me?*

The sweet spot between letting go and directing

Every year at Christmas, when it's time for my family to put up the Christmas tree, I get out the boxes of decorations that have been sitting in a cupboard for the last 11 months. This is often a moment of great excitement for us and the kids, who are eager to dive into the boxes to rediscover the random selection of baubles, lights, and other treats in there. This is also a moment of great stress for me when I realise that the string-lights for the tree will be tangled up. They are either still in a tangle from me trying to pack things away too quickly the year before or are soon to be tangled from the excited rush that is now under way to get things out of storage for this year. The stressful realisation for me is that I will have to spend the next hour or two untangling a long string of lights before we can even start with any tree decoration. Over the years, untangling Christmas tree lights has become one of my least favourite chores, but one of my favourite metaphors for dealing with struggles. Let me explain ...

When faced with a big mess of tangled lights, you have two options: You can either try a very *intentional and controlled* approach of carefully directing one end of the string through various knots and loops, or you can try a very *open to chance* approach of shaking and jiggling the whole string in the hope that it will somehow self-organise into a nice straight line. With the first option, you might successfully manage to navigate the end bulb through one or two loops, but it's not long before you hit a snag and can't go any further. The more you try to force it further in that same direction, the more tightly knotted and entrenched the light tangle becomes. However, if you take the other route of just randomly shaking the whole string in the hope that they will spontaneously self-organise, that won't get you very far either. Indeed, there can be a major risk of this making the situation a whole lot worse – the more shaking you do, the more you lose any sense of direction and control. You may lose all sense of where to start, of which end is which, or whether there's just one knot or now multiple knots in the string. On its own, either option just seems to create more problems.

So, over the years, I've developed a *half-and-half* technique – a third option – where I do a bit of gentle jiggling, just so see what new possibilities arise spontaneously, followed by a bit of intentional directing. Then when I hit a snag, I do another little jiggle to see what happens, then another intentional guide. Another jiggle. Another guide. And so on. I'm not over-controlling the process, nor am I leaving it entirely up to chance. I'm doing both. It's a back-and-forth process between me and the lights, where half of the time I am trusting the lights to do a bit of getting themselves out of this mess, and the other half is me offering a bit of my own intentional input, direction, and help. In both stages – the jiggling and the directing stages – I am trying my best to keep my hands steady, calm, and gentle. Not grabbing or forcing. Of course, this is hard – as more time passes and more stress builds (and the more the kids are getting impatient), the more my own steadiness and patience is tested. But something I've learnt over many years of trying is that rushing or forcing this process is most likely going to backfire. The best chance I have of untangling these lights is by staying calm, patient, and grounded. Keeping my hands gentle and combining a bit of light jiggling with a bit of light-touch direction and guidance. My hands are facilitators of a process, not imposers.

As I write this, I am also reminded of a Chinese finger trap, which is a little tube traditionally made from woven bamboo, designed so you can place a finger in either end. If you try to free your fingers from the trap by pulling them out, the trap tightens, and your fingers become more trapped. The harder you pull, the tighter it gets. It's only when you push your fingers in the opposite direction – almost as though you were giving into, or *relaxing into*, the trap – that it loosens, and you can easily free your fingers.

For me, there are similar themes and lessons involved with negotiating finger traps as there are with negotiating tangled Christmas tree lights: for example, the importance of not forcing it, but relaxing into it. A little bit of direction, combined with a little bit of letting go and being open to trusting in the process. Maybe having a general sense of where you want to end up but not being too predictive and pre-emptive of what the exact path looks like. Not having it all worked out in advance and instead having a willingness to discover new things and find new routes as you go.

To help bring these ideas together, I have sketched a doodle called "holding the tension of the opposites". You may remember earlier in the book I included a "tug-of-war" doodle (page 35), which showed a competitive struggle taking place between two polarised positions. In tug-of-war, the idea is that each of the opposing teams is trying to win. To beat the other one. But this is not the only way of being with two polarised positions. What if both positions had some value? For example, let's say the two positions were *certainty* and *uncertainty*. What if both had something to offer? Sometimes we might want the comfort of certainty, but other times might want the thrill or challenge of uncertainty. Also, we might find that too much certainty would be stagnating, whereas too much uncertainty would be disorientating. So we don't want one to win over the other. We want both. We want balance.

In this doodle, I am offering the idea of transitioning from a *tug-of-war* scenario into a *see-saw*! So rather than competitively pulling to overcome the other, we are instead playfully moving between the two. A bit of certainty can help us to lay the foundation to embrace some novelty and change. Also, a bit of uncertainty can help us grow and expand ourselves and get a broader understanding of who we are. There is a balance here. These are two opposing positions, but they are working together in a way where one can help the other out. On a see-saw, having two opposing positions is not only more pleasurable for both parties, but a necessity for the system to work at all.

HOLDING THE TENSION OF THE OPPOSITES

① TUG-OF-WAR

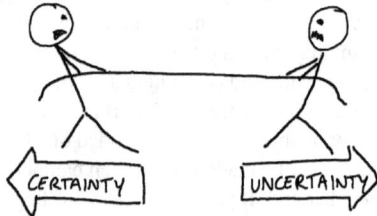

CERTAINTY   UNCERTAINTY

② HELD GENTLY

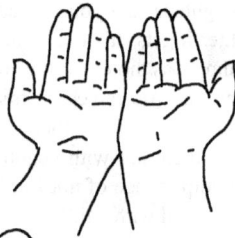

③ SEE-SAW

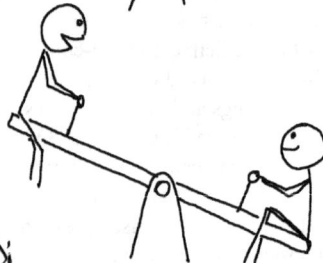

The difference between CONTROLLING uncertainty, holding the tension, and playfully moving in and out of uncertainty.

DOODLE: "Holding the tension of the opposites"

With my Christmas tree lights, there is a back-and-forth movement between 'directing' and 'letting go'. Directing ... letting go ... directing ... letting go. And all the while this process is being held gently in a pair of hands. We can think of these hands as the compassionate self – the 'third person' position, just holding, caring, overseeing, and guiding the process.

Learning safe ways to let go of control

We have already established that letting go of control will inevitably involve emotions. This might be feelings of stress, fear, and vulnerability. Your certainty-seeking brain will be giving you these emotions to tell you that you are entering into unfamiliar territory – into novelty and unpredictability. Your brain's emotions are not telling you that you're doing anything wrong or bad. They are not there to judge you, nor to punish you. They are there to tell you that you are entering into the places *around the edges* of certainty. They are also a reminder that if you do indeed want to go there, then it might be helpful to equip yourself with a particular stance: a mindset ready for exploration, not control; a body ready for courage, not comfort; an intention for growth and expansion, not for maintenance and protection.

If you have ever tried a so-called "trust fall" – which is where you allow yourself to fall backwards and trust that the other person will catch you – you might have a sense of the emotional stages involved. Perhaps there is a strong initial spike of fear as you are about to start your fall. This may be followed by a surrendering of control, and a feeling of *letting go* as you hand over your full trust to the other person. There is courage involved in starting the movement – to navigate the initial spike of fear – as well as a wisdom and trust in knowing that it will be okay on the other side. Maybe this is a person you know and who you can rely on. Once these pillars of courage, wisdom, and trust are all in place, you may be able to embrace the experience of letting go, and perhaps even enjoy it. While the idea of *surrender* might be terrifying for those of us who have always tended to rely on control in the past, under the right circumstances, this can be highly liberating. In this section, we will consider some of the ways that humans have found ways to embrace surrender and letting go as a step towards positive transformation and growth.

In a thesis I wrote 20 years ago, while studying in London for a Master's degree in *Psychology of Religion*, I reviewed some of the literature on spiritual and mystical experiences, as well as on other altered states of consciousness. (This work was subsequently published in 2008 in the journal, *Mental Health, Religion, and Culture* [63]). Part of this paper involved describing mystical experiences in terms of both a "self-surrender" stage, where there is a breakdown of existing cognitive (or self) structures, and a "new vision" stage, which involves transcending these old cognitive structures to reveal new meaning [64]. A main focus of the thesis was to highlight how similar processes of ego breakdown and restructuring can occur in very different contexts – from religion and spirituality, to recreational drug use, to the clinical contexts of trauma, dissociation, and psychosis. Sometimes this process can be transformational. Sometimes it can be distressing and disruptive. In religious contexts, self-surrender can be facilitated through a range of intentional practices and rituals such as fasting, sensory deprivation, and chanting, as well as through meditative practice and prayer. Psychoactive drugs, particularly psychedelics, can be taken by people who want to chemically stimulate these kinds of processes. In trauma and psychosis, as I was arguing, there may often be similar processes occurring, albeit in a less intentional way. In other words, a less controlled entry into these spaces of losing control.

These early academic interests of mine have led to many subsequent years of reading, learning about, and studying these areas – for example, investigating and writing about: the overlap between spiritual and psychotic experiences; the effects of drugs on the human brain (especially drugs that have dissociative or psychedelic properties); the effects of traumatic experience on the brain and mind; dissociation; the concept of post-traumatic growth. As a clinical academic and self-help author, I have also been passionately focused on how to help people who are struggling with their past traumas and threat-patterns to move towards compassionate understanding and integration, and ultimately to transformation and growth.

As *Controlled Explosions* is a book written for all of us – a general audience, as opposed to an academic and research audience, I have tried to keep the scientific issues and research questions mostly to one side. We have focused primarily on the lived experience of controlled explosions and the relevance to our daily lives. So, this would not be a good point, as we enter the latter stages of the book, to start bombarding you with scientific studies. I instead want to stay in the spirit of self-experience and self-understanding by sharing with you a couple of other book recommendations that explore, in an accessible way, the subjects we are touching on here – losing control and post-traumatic growth. The books are *The Art of Losing Control* [65] and *When You're Falling, Dive* [43], which are listed along with some other recommended resources in Appendix 5. In *The Art of Losing Control*, philosopher Jules Evans documents some of the historical ways that humans have attempted to achieve self-transcendence (such as through religion, art, dance, music, sex, meditation, psychedelic drugs, war, and so on). He argues that ecstatic experiences have always been sought after and are important for our human flourishing and growth. In the other book, *When You're Falling, Dive*, Mark Matousek interviews people about the transformational experiences they have been through after a major crisis or trauma in their life. There are some inspiring accounts of how people can embrace the change process that may occur after crisis.

There's vitality in facing life's extremes, including that of your own extinction. Crises pushes you to travel wide, fast and deep, expands the heart and calls forth reserves of courage you didn't know you had, like adrenaline in the muscles of a mother saving her only child. Only you are the child, and it's your life – the life of your own soul – that you are saving.

(Mark Matousek [43])

One thing I have taken from reading these books, as well as through my own studies and work in this area, is that our brains can – and do – go through powerful transformational processes. Our perceptual frameworks are not fixed, nor are the neural circuits wired to support them. These frameworks can be reconfigured and updated. The neural circuits can be rewired. Neuroplasticity – the constant wiring and rewiring of our brain's neural circuits – is a lifelong process, and is something we can all embrace, rather than resist. If I didn't believe that brains could heal and change, I wouldn't have spent the last 20 years being a therapist and setting up a therapy centre.

The processes of transformation and growth typically involve a breaking-down or letting-go of an old framework – an old version of ourselves and way of organising our lives – and in its place rebuilding a new structure and new version of ourselves. Sometimes this process can be actively sought after (and has been throughout human history). Sometimes this process is thrust upon us due to something major that has happened in our life, which demands a new version of us to emerge. In both cases, the transformation process can come with potential rewards as well as potential risks. It can be enriching or destabilising and because of the scary and destabilising elements, many of us will resist it. We might feel safer to stay with the familiarity of the old version of ourselves, and with controlled explosions that keep the old fears and old circuits intact.

HARM CREATED: *Entering into a place of vulnerability alongside feared emotions*

GROWTH OPENED: *Building a new structure better suited for the future*

Bringing it all together

In this book, we have learnt about many different examples of *controlled explosions* that can occur in our lives. These were introduced to us as 15 members of the bomb squad, along with three key pieces of kit they can use in creating controlled explosions. To help us understand the various functions of controlled explosions, we personified the explosion-creators as characters, each with specific objectives. Their objectives and methods were all slightly different but shared the common theme of being threat-focused, in that they were protecting us from bigger harms that they feared and predicted might happen. Throughout these chapters we used a simple two-part template to help us identify and map out these protective functions, in terms of **HARM CREATED** and **HARM AVERTED**. With more of an understanding of the function of our controlled explosions, we were in a better position to make a wise (informed) choice about whether to accept it, whether to address it (and its causes/fears), or whether to switch to a different strategy for avoiding these underlying fears. These choices are laid out in a more systematic way for you in Appendix 3.

In this chapter, we have ventured into exploring more what the "address" option might look like. As we emphasised, all three options (accept, address, and switch) are all equally valid. While this book has aimed to help you map out and understand your choices, only you know what choice is right for you, and when. This chapter has provided some ideas for a path we can take if we did want to address the underlying fears that are driving controlled explosions. The first step involved a collaborative process of discovery with the bomb squad members – working with them, rather than against them or in conflict with them. We uncovered that often our averted harms can be linked to past threats and traumas in our lives, and to basic needs we had as younger versions of ourselves. These needs may have been unmet, or they may have been thwarted or threatened in some way. Hence, through this collaborative process of discovery with the bomb squad we were able to link the functions of our controlled explosions (the **HARM AVERTED**) with some crucial information about ourselves, our fears, and our basic needs.

From inner controllers to inner allies

We have recognised the role of compassion – and specifically our compassionate self – in helping us to navigate the process of engaging and dialoguing with our bomb squad members. We found that this process, if approached with care and compassion, could guide us closer to finding out what these harms are, and what needs they are rooted in. We were able to understand that the reason we are avoiding/averting these things is because they are so painful, and the reason they are so painful is because they are interwoven with our fundamental needs. Connecting with this material is hard. It takes courage, time, and tolerance. It involves holding the tension, being with it, and leaning into it. We considered why compassionate leaning into, rather than moving away from, would be the ideal formula not only for how we relate to the hurt, vulnerable, and needy parts of us, but also for how we relate to the bomb squad more generally. Rather than seeing them simply as inner controllers and threat-protectors, stuck in patterns of repeating harm towards us, we can start to appreciate their potential role as collaborators and allies in holding key information about ourselves. We noted that this doesn't mean we would necessarily choose the bomb squad to be our most wise and helpful teachers or friends. (Remember they are linked to brain states rooted in our threat system, and do not have specific motivations towards us – to either care or harm). But neither should we dismiss them, fight them, reject, or silence them. They have specialist knowledge about our deepest fears, threats, and traumas. And this information is key for identifying our needs – both the (unmet) needs that we can let go of from the past, as well as the needs that we can start to build our life around in the future.

Here I have brought these elements together as a visual summary.

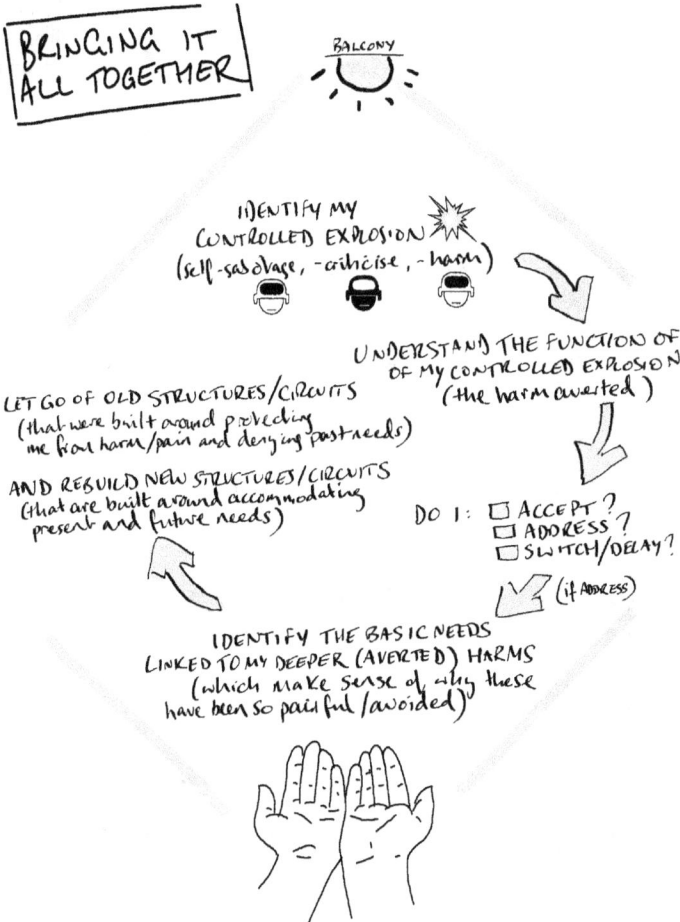

DOODLE: "Bringing it all together"

One of our main discoveries about your bomb squad is that they have been working tirelessly to protect an old structure – a past version of you. One that was designed and built around the imperative to not re-experience the pain of a past wound. The *controlled explosions* have been protecting you on the assumption that you must keep this old structure intact and stop it from be-coming over-loaded – for example, to prevent any build-up of pressure, energy, emotional tension that might destabilise or break it. But what if, as we have been asking in this chapter, the structure itself was outdated and no longer fit for purpose? What if the old structure or circuit simply cannot (and can never) accommodate the life experiences, needs, and the emotional range that you re-quire of it now? A bit like the old bridge that can no longer accommodate the new volume of traffic. Perhaps there are moments in life when we all must accept that our old brain circuits can no longer accommodate the full range of emotions, perceptions, and actions that are required for our changing worlds.

Even though the old structure may have served you well in the past, new struc-tures may now be required for new circumstances – structures that will allow you to *outgrow* your fears, rather than avoid them. This is where the processes of letting go and rebuilding can happen. Breaking down the old structure and wel-coming in the new. On page 135, I gave examples of some of the places I might look for replacing an old (younger) version of Charlie with a new version. What would this look like for you? What would be the old versions of you, linked to past threats, that are ready to be updated? Don't worry if you're not quite sure yet. It may be that insights will emerge for you over time. And remember the imagery exercises I've included, such as meeting your younger self and your future self, will be there for you to come back to at any time, and as many times as you need.

From threat-protecting to growth-expanding controlled explosions

THREAT AND PROTECTION FOCUSED:

HARM AVERTED: Attack and reject myself

HARM CREATED: Avoid being vulnerable to experience of rejection from others

⬇

NEEDS IDENTIFIED:
Connecting to others and belonging

⬆

GROWTH AND EXPANSION FOCUSED:

HARM CREATED: Entering vulnerability and holding the tension of painful emotions

GROWTH OPENED: New structure that accomodates an expanded range of emotions

Transformation and growth, as we have learnt, are longer-lasting solutions to *controlled explosions*, as they address their causes and functions. If you choose to no longer accept *controlled explosions*, nor to switch over to alternatives, then addressing and resolving them may be a good choice for you. Addressing them is not about getting rid of the bomb squad, it is about resolving and outgrowing the fears at the root of why they are there in the first place. This involves courageously holding the tension, resisting the urge to control, until you can see clearly into what fears, threats, traumas, and needs are behind them.

It involves replacing threat with safeness and replacing conflict with compassion. It involves letting go of unmet needs from the past and replacing them with needs and wants for the future. It involves replacing old brain circuits that excluded emotions and needs with new *expanded* circuits that can include them. It involves redirecting energy resources away from controlling and maintaining the old patterns, towards building up new ones. These are the kinds of transformations that will show your bomb squad that *controlled explosions* are no longer required, and that it is safe for the new version of you to start showing up in your life.

In conclusion

This book has explored a complex area of our psychological lives which is equally as intriguing as it is troublesome. Many of us are caught in self-defeating patterns, and while our societies and mental health industries seem more intent on finding ways to help us numb and avoid these, this book has taken a deep dive into uncovering the complexities of why they might be happening. Leaning into this complexity has required us to first let go of the idea that our brain should work perfectly for us, and that when it doesn't, something must be wrong. Our brain does *not* work perfectly. And this does *not* mean something is wrong. Our brain is a survival machine. It is programmed not to optimise our happiness and well-being, but to keep us alive. It needs us to exist in a predictable world. It does not like surprises. It does not want us to be caught off guard. It shapes our perceptions and directs our actions away from encountering such vulnerabilities; avoiding what may be detrimental to survival. Being exposed to threats and dangers is bad enough, but the most vulnerable state for us humans is being exposed to *unpredictable* threat. Our brain cannot allow this, and will intervene to give us more controlled, predictable versions of threat. Our brain would rather we were the arbiter of our own downfall than risk being floored by something external. It would rather we were well-rehearsed in receiving internally-created hostility than risk being unprepared for it from others. Controlled explosions are doing a job for us. They harm us, yes. But they keep this harm in-house, at controlled levels, as part of a complex trade-off where the alternative may be a harm that totally overwhelms us.

Addressing your brain's self-destructive patterns is unlikely to ever be a case of simple solutions and quick fixes. These are driven by processes linked to underlying fears, conflicts, and traumas from your personal life that are still waiting for the right moment to be seen, understood, and resolved. Opening your mind to the early origins of your self-sabotage takes time and care. It also takes courage. It is a tough choice, but potentially one of the most self-compassionate choices you could ever make. It's a decision to turn towards vulnerability, not away from it. To accept that you have valid needs, as well as very real hurts, fears, grievances, and losses around those needs. To be committed to caring for these hurt parts of you and finding ways to accommodate and welcome them into the new structures of your life. The choice is to defuse controlled explosions with compassion.

Appendices

Appendix 1

Background and how I came into the metaphor

My background influences

Many of the ideas in this book are influenced by the model I have been most drawn to in my life as a practising mental health professional, Compassion Focused Therapy (CFT). The founder of CFT, Paul Gilbert, has been an enormous influence on my approach to communicating concepts around brains and mental health. Gilbert typically starts his lectures and presentations with a joke, and much of his communication of ideas uses playful, light-hearted language, often with metaphors and stories. For example, the language of 'tricky brains' is directly from Gilbert and CFT. As is the language of 'loops' and 'multiple selves' (angry self, anxious self, sad self, and self-critic). The metaphors and playful language not only help create a warm and affiliative tone, but crucially, from a CFT perspective, they also help with de-shaming a lot of these experiences and struggles for people. If you approach your well-being and suffering from a position of shame, it's going to be much harder to bring a helpful and caring orientation in your efforts to be helpful.

The other major influence behind the ideas in this book is Carl Jung. My thinking about psychology was heavily shaped by Jung's ideas long before Gilbert or any other influences, dating back from first reading *Memories, Dreams, Reflections* as a teenager, and then through studying *Jung and the Post-Jungians* for a MA degree in Psychology of Religion in my early twenties. I was writing essays on Jung's theory of archetypal psychology before I had even started my career in mental health, prior to starting Clinical Psychology training at the age of 27. It is fair to say that Jung's influence is not so much on the light-hearted side! Indeed, his writings are often very complex, obscure, and confusing. And yet utterly ground-breaking and transformative. I would say Jung's main influence on me is how he views mental activity through the lens of uncovering its underlying function. What's in the engine-room behind mental events. With religion, for example, Jung posits an innate religious function within the human psyche that we are all born with. So, regardless of whether religious ideas and beliefs are rational (or 'true', as it were), human beings are still *naturally* religious (for a reason) – i.e., having religious beliefs serves our species in some way. Similarly, with dreams, fantasies, illusions, art, and so on, Jung is interested in looking *behind* these – at what are the archetypal (inherited) patterns in our minds that organise and structure these mental activities.

Jung taught me to be curious about *why* mental patterns exist. Even if, on the surface, some mental phenomena and processes may be highly irrational, illogical, and often outright unhelpful, there may be some underlying process that – at some level – is valid, meaningful, and functional. This curiosity has guided a lot of my clinical work, particularly in developing and providing therapies for people with psychosis who experience distressing voices and beliefs (the subject of my previous book, *Relating to Voices*). To me, I can never be satisfied with writing off someone's lived experience as a meaningless 'pathology' or an aberrant mis-firing neuron. I am always curious as to *why* this is happening. What's driving this? If not the surface level, then at what level – in the background engine room of the mind – do we need to explore to find the valid expression, meaning, or function?

As well as the Gilbert and Jung influences behind this book, there other many other original and novel ideas that are presented here for the first time. These are not emerging from CFT or Jungian Psychology perspectives, but from my own personal journals that I've been writing for 25 years, as I have grappled with the day-to-day struggles of my own mental health, those of my family, friends, colleagues, and importantly the many hundreds of clients I have had the privilege of learning from in the therapy room.

My story into developing and using the metaphor

For many years, I have been intrigued by the various ways in which our minds work that are harmful and destructive to us, and I have been trying to make sense of this for myself and for the people who have come to me for help. In a 2008 paper entitled *Mysticism and Madness*, I was considering how an evolutionary understanding might help us to make sense of why inherited traits associated with psychosis-related conditions like schizophrenia still exist in our gene pool and have not been removed by natural selection. If these conditions are so harmful and detrimental to our functioning and survival, why do they endure? In what ways could these possibly be of benefit to us? An evolutionary functional analysis helps us to make sense of these things because the traits and characteristics that we inherit through evolutionary processes typically come as a trade-off, i.e. there may be advantages (such as to survival) of having a certain trait, but also this trait may disadvantage us in other ways.

> *Thus, the reason why schizotypy has not been 'ejected' by natural selection must be that it actually benefits our species in a different way, and that the selective advantage of these beneficial effects must counteract the selective*

disadvantage of psychosis ... The point is that schizotypal personality is
actually useful, and to enjoy its benefits, we unfortunately must suffer its
most extreme consequences from time to time. [63].

Although a psychological trait or process may be harmful to us (as individuals), there may be other benefits that are perhaps less obvious, and which
may not even benefit us at the individual level at all, but more at a collective
(species) level. There are countless examples of evolutionary trade-offs, and
when it comes to evolved mental processes, often the trade-off is that we
inherit emotions and processes that are very good at enhancing our protection
and survival, but which, unfortunately, have a considerable negative impact
on our mental health.

The overarching concept here – that the same thing can be both harmful
(in one context) and helpful (in another context) – can be tricky to understand,
and something that I have tried to explain many times to people (sometimes
repeatedly, and often without much success!). I've attempted to explain this
concept to clients in therapy sessions, to clinicians attending workshops, as
well as to academics in journal articles and peer reviews. It's not an easy concept to communicate or grasp, and perhaps its complexity comes from the ap-
parent contradiction: having to hold two competing 'truths' in mind. How can
something be both harmful and helpful at the same time? It doesn't follow our
usual rules of logic. A few years ago, I was questioned on exactly this point by
a journal editor as part of the peer review process for an academic article on
voice-hearing. The editor was not convinced about the idea that there could
be some function or advantage in the experience of hearing critical voices:

"What is the utility of entering into a painful and consuming talk with ma-
levolent voice? Seems that the cost largely exceeds the pros."
(Journal editor, 2021)

It is no surprise that it takes a while for people to get their heads around
this. To navigate the contradiction requires us to simultaneously hold two contexts in mind – one in which something is harmful (an individual context) and
another in which it is helpful (an evolutionary context). The mental gymnas-
tics required highlights the clear need for a good metaphor!

Metaphors help us to understand complex ideas by drawing a parallel with
something that we are familiar with. So this got me contemplating about what
might be some parallels? What familiar examples are there of things that are
both harmful and helpful? The common phrase 'cruel to be kind' comes to
mind, although this is not something I have ever liked personally. For me, this
evokes something similar to how a parent may want to 'teach them a lesson' to
their child, and even though the parent's motivation may be caring, and they
may strongly believe this will actually help their child – "it's for their own

good" – this is often not what it feels like for the child receiving this. The idea of 'tough love' may be in a similar ballpark.

These were not quite right for what I needed the metaphor to do. I was aware that this style of parenting is now seen by many as outdated, and research studies have demonstrated that the long-term consequences of this may not actually be as helpful as the parents had believed or intended. Nor did it quite fit with the message of the 'Compassionate Parenting' course that I was working on at the time! (with an Educational Psychologist colleague, Jo Taylor [66]). I needed a metaphor that conveyed something clearly harm-making in one context, and yet genuinely (and *indisputably*) helpful in another context.

I came to realise that if you contemplate a problem for long enough, then eventually a creative solution will jump out at you. And the metaphor I was looking for jumped out at me from a very unexpected place – a crime thriller series on TV! I arrived at the metaphor of controlled explosions while watching the British TV series, *Trigger Point* [67], which stars Vicky McClure as a bomb disposal expert who heads up a Police bomb squad. The episodes of this series, first aired in January 2022, show the bomb squad having to use various techniques for disabling bombs and keeping the public safe from harm. Many of the techniques involved some kind of controlled explosion, where the bomb is detonated or disabled in a contained, controlled way that minimises the greater harm that would occur from an out-of-control blast.

Unlike 'cruel to be kind', this metaphor has the benefit of being something we can all agree is genuinely helpful. Another benefit is that bombs and explosions are things we are all familiar with from our TV shows, as well as from the news. In the UK, *Trigger Point* was ranked in the Top 10 most-watched programmes of the whole year (and for UK viewers, 2022 was not short of major TV events, from the FIFA football World Cup[1] to the State Funeral of Queen Elizabeth II [68]).

The 'controlled explosions' metaphor certainly fitted the remit of what I required, so the next step was to see how this metaphor landed when applied to the lived experiences of people struggling with their mental health. This is exactly what I've been testing out over the last three years since 2022, in my writing/journalling, teaching, and in my therapy practice. I have found that this metaphor can really help people to develop a non-shaming understanding about their own self-destructive patterns and self-inflicted harms. The controlled explosion metaphor has now become successfully incorporated into my clinical, teaching, and academic work, and this was one of the big motivators for writing this book. Not only did I want to share this metaphor more widely to help more people, but I also wanted to use it to hold together and structure the chapters of this book so that you, the reader, would have a clear and consistent framework for exploring this important topic with me.

SELF DEFEAT
— AN EVOLUTIONARY STRATEGY TO PROTECT US FROM THE PAIN OF BEING DEFEATED / THWARTED BY EXTERNAL EVENTS OUT OF OUR CONTROL

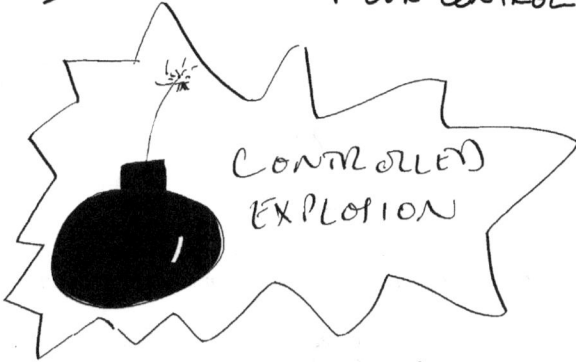

CONTROLLED EXPLOSION

KEEP IT 'IN HOUSE'
— often the least-worst option

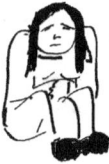

• Self-inflict the pain now before someone / thing else does
• Self-inflict pain as a preparatory measure (to increase your general tolerance to / mastery over pain)

DOODLE: "Self-defeat" (my very first doodle when developing the metaphor)

Note

1 Speaking of football, I'm reminded of the old military proverb that we regularly hear from sports commentators: 'attack is the best form of defence'!

Appendix 2

The Transpersonal Experiences Questionnaire

The *Transpersonal Experiences Questionnaire* (TEQ) [69]. Reproduced with permission.

1 *have you had the experience of suddenly feeling as if you were in contact with someone who is not physically present, or knowing what they were thinking or feeling?*
2 *have you had the experience of seeing something that other people couldn't see, or that you later found out was not there?*
3 *have you had the experience of your thoughts being read or picked up by other people?*
4 *have you had the experience of smelling something that other people are not aware of, or that is only perceptible to you?*
5 *have you had the experience of thoughts rushing very rapidly through your mind, so that one idea after another comes into your head and the thoughts seem to whirl around beyond your control?*
6 *have you had the experience of some kind of 'mission' or duty being revealed to you, and knowing that you have to fulfil this mission, or feeling compelled to do so?*
7 *have you had experiences of unusual sensations in your body, not created by any obvious physical cause, for example of heat or cold, energy moving, or something entering or passing through your body?*
8 *have you had experiences in which things in the world around you seemed to contain messages or hints, perhaps in a metaphorical or symbolic way?*
9 *have you had the experience of picking up on other people's thoughts?*
10 *have you had the experience of feeling monitored or watched, or otherwise the subject of external attention, when there is no obvious cause for this?*

11 *have you had the experience of feeling emotions or thinking thoughts that were actually those of other people?*

12 *have you experienced being in a state in which you felt cut off or isolated from things and people around you, perhaps as if there were some invisible barrier around you that prevented a normal connection?*

13 *have you had the experience of observing an event happen and feeling as though you had caused it with your mind?*

14 *have you had the experience of disorientation in time, so that for example, the past and the future seem distant or unavailable, and the present moment dominates, or time seems to lose its meaning?*

15 *have you experienced your bodily movements being controlled by someone or something outside of you?*

16 *have you had an experience of having your thoughts, feelings or movements influenced by other people's thoughts or gestures?*

17 *have you had an experience of a loss of your individual identity and a sense of being part of some greater whole that extends far beyond you?*

18 *have you had the experience of hearing things, like voices talking, when there hasn't been anyone around?*

19 *have you had the experience of feeling as though events in your environment, such as the actions or comments of other people, are in reference to you, or are directed at you, even though you know that this is unlikely?*

Appendix 3

Controlled explosion worksheets

Appendices **3.1** to **3.15** are a collection of worksheets that you can use for mapping out your own controlled explosions, and for then thinking about what choices you have.

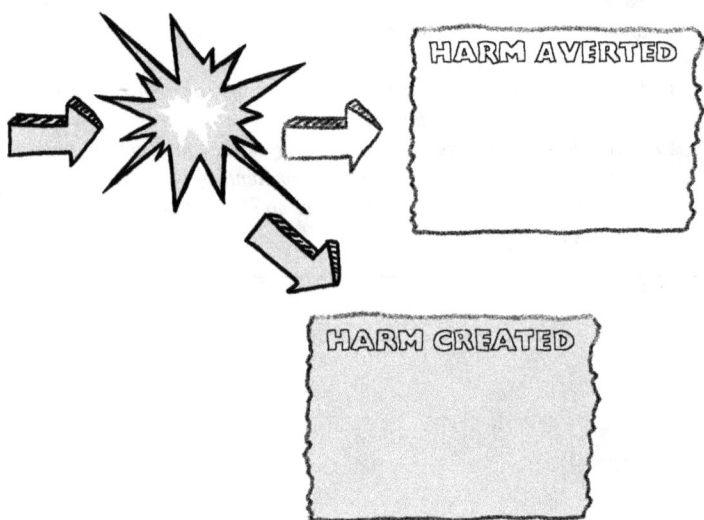

Once you've identified a controlled explosion in your life, and mapped it out (in terms of **HARM CREATED** and **AVERTED**, there's three main choices and options of what you can do:

ACCEPT: Go along with the controlled explosion, knowing you've made a choice to accept the sabotage/harm that it's creating, in service of averting another harm

ADDRESS: Address the fear that the controlled explosion is protecting you from (the harm averted) so that use of controlled explosions is less necessary

SWITCH/DELAY: If you're not ready (yet) to address the fear itself, then seeing if there is an alternative controlled explosion that is less harmful to use (for now).

Appendices **3.1** to **3.15** provide illustrative examples for all 15 members of the bomb squad of the difference between an 'accept', 'address' or 'switch/delay' choice. Each one is followed by a blank table for you to work through if you have your own example of this.

It is important for us to realise we do have choices. Even through these controlled explosions might have been (unconscious) creations of our brain – things that we did not choose – now that we are aware of them, we do have choices. These worksheet examples give an initial taster of what these choices might be, but see Chapter 6 for further guidance on the 'address' option – what it may look like choosing to address the roots of these controlled explosions.

Appendix 3.1   Self-sabotage unit: CERTAINTY-SEEKER

SITUATION: I want a career change, but the first job I applied to in the new field never got back to me, so I'm concluding the career must not be right for me and giving up on the idea

I've identified that my **CERTAINTY-SEEKER** is creating this controlled explosion:

> **HARM CREATED:** *giving up on the idea of a career change*

> **HARM AVERTED:** *avoiding the experience of uncertainty*

Do I accept this? Do I want to address it? Or switch to a different strategy?

ACCEPT: Yes, I do want to stop these uncomfortable feelings of uncertainty by dropping the idea of a different career

ADDRESS: No, I don't want to let go of this idea, and yet I can see that my brain is struggling with feelings of uncertainty. To address this, I will intentionally prepare myself and my body to tolerate some uncomfortable feelings as I keep pushing forward and find out what will come of this

SWITCH/DELAY: Yes, I do want to reduce the feeling of uncertainty, but rather than giving up on the idea, I am instead going to contact the job to see if they received my application and if they can provide any feedback

YOUR EXAMPLE. Self-sabotage unit: CERTAINTY SEEKER

SITUATION:

I've identified that my **CERTAINTY-SEEKER** is creating this controlled explosion:

> **HARM CREATED:** ...

> **HARM AVERTED:** ...

Do I accept this? Do I want to address it? Or switch to a different strategy?

ACCEPT:

ADDRESS:

SWITCH/DELAY:

Appendix 3.2   Self-sabotage unit: PROCRASTINATOR

SITUATION: I am trying to focus on writing a book, but I keep reaching for my phone to check if there are any new notifications

I've identified that my **PROCRASTINATOR** is creating this controlled explosion:

> **HARM CREATED:** *seeking a novel experience/sensation outside of the task*
>
> **HARM AVERTED:** *avoiding the experience of task monotony*

Do I accept this? Do I want to address it? Or switch to a different strategy?

ACCEPT: Yes, I do want to take my mind away from the monotony of this task by seeking something new and exciting on my phone

ADDRESS: No, I don't want to take my mind away from the task, and yet I can see that my brain is struggling with monotony and has an urge for something new and exciting. To address this, I will try to make the task itself more exciting and less monotonous by setting myself a challenge like writing one paragraph in 10 minutes. *How about writing some of this book in a weird font? That creates a bit of novelty!* Will that font make it through the publishing process I wonder?

SWITCH/DELAY: Yes, I do want to take my mind away from the monotony of this task, but rather than seeking something new and exciting on my phone, I am instead going to take a break and come back to it when I'm feeling refreshed

---

YOUR EXAMPLE. Self-sabotage unit: PROCRASTINATOR

SITUATION:

I've identified that my **PROCRASTINATOR** is creating this controlled explosion:

HARM CREATED: ...

HARM AVERTED: ...

Do I accept this? Do I want to address it? Or switch to a different strategy?

ACCEPT:

ADDRESS:

SWITCH/DELAY:

Appendix 3.3 Self-sabotage unit: PERFECTIONIST

SITUATION: I am writing an important email to my boss, but I keep going back over and double-checking and rewriting each sentence multiple times

I've identified that my **PERFECTIONIST** is creating this controlled explosion:

> **HARM CREATED:** *I am rigorously error-checking against an impossible standard*

> **HARM AVERTED:** *Fear of making an error, failure, and possibly criticism/ punishment*

Do I accept this? Do I want to address it? Or switch to a different strategy?

ACCEPT: Yes, I do want to avoid feeling that fear, and am willing to keep checking over this email and getting it more and more perfect with tweaks and changes for as long as it takes

ADDRESS: No, I don't want to spend more hours on this email, and yet I can see that my brain is caught in a pattern of fear. To address this, I will investigate what the fear is about, notice where this feeling is in my body, take a deep breath into that and tell myself that it will be okay

SWITCH/DELAY: Yes, I do want to avoid the fear feeling, but rather than spending more and more hours on this same email now, I will instead save the draft and come back to it another day (credit: **PROCRASTINATOR**)

YOUR EXAMPLE. Self-sabotage unit: PERFECTIONIST

SITUATION:

I've identified that my **PERFECTIONIST** is creating this controlled explosion:

> **HARM CREATED:** ...

> **HARM AVERTED:** ...

Do I accept this? Do I want to address it? Or switch to a different strategy?

ACCEPT:

ADDRESS:

SWITCH/DELAY:

Appendix 3.4   Self-sabotage unit: PESSIMIST

SITUATION: I am with my friends at the beach, and they start to play
a game of beach cricket. I have never played cricket
before and assume it will end up badly, so I don't join
in

I've identified that my **PESSIMIST** is creating this controlled explosion:

> **HARM CREATED:** *I'm not going to join in playing this game because I'll be
bad at it*
>
> **HARM AVERTED:** *Fear of failure and experiencing shame and
embarrassment*

Do I accept this? Do I want to address it? Or switch to a different strategy?

ACCEPT: Yes, I do want to avoid the possibility of failure at all
costs, and I am willing to sabotage any potential
enjoyment I might get from joining in this game

ADDRESS: No, I don't want to miss out on the pleasure and fun
that I could have with my friends, and yet I can see
that my brain is stuck in predicting my failure and
humiliation. To address this, I will recognise that these
fear predictions are linked to a difficult experience
that happened to me at school when I was younger,
and remind myself that a lot has changed since
school-days

SWITCH/DELAY: Yes, I do want to avoid the fear of failure, but instead
of sabotaging my own pleasure by not joining, I will
instead sabotage the quality of the game by joining in
with intentionally wild and silly shots so everyone can
see that I'm just messing around

YOUR EXAMPLE. Self-sabotage unit: PESSIMIST

SITUATION:

I've identified that my **PESSIMIST** is creating this controlled explosion:

> **HARM CREATED:** ...
>
> **HARM AVERTED:** ...

Do I accept this? Do I want to address it? Or switch to a different strategy?

ACCEPT:

ADDRESS:

SWITCH/DELAY:

Appendix 3.5   Self-sabotage unit: CHAOS-CREATOR

SITUATION: I am stuck in indecision about my career. I am not enjoying my job, but at the same time I'm scared about leaving because of paying the bills. I'm desperate to not make the wrong decision

I've identified that my **CHAOS-CREATOR** is creating this controlled explosion:

> **HARM CREATED:** *I create a problem at work that speeds up my decision to leave*
>
> **HARM AVERTED:** *Crippling indecision about my job*

Do I accept this? Do I want to address it? Or switch to a different strategy?

ACCEPT: Yes, I do want to stop this uncomfortable feeling of indecision and the fear of getting it wrong, and creating a 'scene' is the most effective way to take the decision out of my hands

ADDRESS: No, I don't want to create drama and problems, and yet I can see that my brain is struggling with the indecision. To address this, I will hold the tension of not knowing for a while and lean in to understanding what the fears are about. Are there other times in my life where I've felt this? I will tune in to how I feel, rather than what is right or wrong, because sometimes in life there is no right or wrong

SWITCH/DELAY: Yes, I do want to stop this feeling of indecision, but rather than creating chaos, I'm going to get my dad to decide for me

---

YOUR EXAMPLE. Self-sabotage unit – CHAOS CREATOR

SITUATION:

I've identified that my **CHAOS-CREATOR** is creating this controlled explosion:

> **HARM CREATED:** ...
>
> **HARM AVERTED:** ...

Do I accept this? Do I want to address it? Or switch to a different strategy?

ACCEPT:

ADDRESS:

SWITCH/DELAY:

Appendix 3.6.   Self-criticism unit: IMPROVER

SITUATION: I am criticising myself for messing things up and I keep
                     highlighting to myself all the ways that I am flawed and
                     inadequate

I've identified that my **IMPROVER** is creating this controlled explosion:

   HARM CREATED: *Pointing out my mistakes, flaws, inadequacies to myself*

   HARM AVERTED: *Other people seeing my mistakes, flaws, and
                     inadequacies*

Do I accept this? Do I want to address it? Or switch to a different strategy?

ACCEPT: Yes, I do want to make sure that my flaws are not seen
                     by others, and staying constantly focused on my own
                     shortcomings is a price worth paying

ADDRESS: No, I don't want to keep focusing on my flaws all the
                     time, and yet I can see that my brain is afraid of
                     letting this go in case this makes me vulnerable to
                     other people's judgements. To address this, I will get
                     to the bottom of why I am so sensitive to people's
                     judgements. Is it linked to something that happened
                     when I was younger?

SWITCH/DELAY: Yes, I do want to make sure that my flaws are
                   not seen by others, but rather than constantly
                   focusing on these, I will call on the services of
                   the **PERFECTIONIST** to make sure that I achieve
                   flawlessness

YOUR EXAMPLE. Self-criticism unit – IMPROVER

SITUATION:

I've identified that my **IMPROVER** is creating this controlled explosion:

   HARM CREATED: ...

   HARM AVERTED: ...

Do I accept this? Do I want to address it? Or switch to a different strategy?

ACCEPT:

ADDRESS:

SWITCH/DELAY:

Appendix 3.7   Self-criticism unit: BLAMER

SITUATION: I have always felt everything is my fault, ever since I was a young child. When I was really young, I wanted my mother to notice me, but she was more interested in that little black rectangle thing with a screen that lights up. It was my fault for not being good enough

I've identified that my **BLAMER** is creating this controlled explosion:

HARM CREATED: *It's my fault that I must not be good/interesting/ important enough*

HARM AVERTED: *Avoid the possibility that my parent might be wrong and that I might be angry about that*

Do I accept this? Do I want to address it? Or switch to a different strategy?

ACCEPT: Yes, I do want to avoid the risk of getting angry and into conflict with others, and I accept that the safest way to do this is by always blaming myself

ADDRESS: No, I don't want to self-blame any more, and yet I can see that my brain is naturally geared towards avoiding anger and confrontation with others. To address this, I can see that while it was understandable that my child 'self' had to develop this strategy, as an adult, things are different, and I can now learn to communicate if I disagree with people, or if I think they are wrong or at fault

SWITCH/DELAY: Yes, I do want to avoid the risk of getting into conflicts with others, but rather than self-blaming all the time, I will instead put my angry energy into complaining about more general things like the world and the government

YOUR EXAMPLE. Self-criticism unit – BLAMER

SITUATION:

I've identified that my **BLAMER** is creating this controlled explosion:

HARM CREATED: ...

HARM AVERTED: ...

Do I accept this? Do I want to address it? Or switch to a different strategy?

ACCEPT:

ADDRESS:

SWITCH/DELAY:

Appendix 3.8   Self-criticism unit: DISCHARGER

SITUATION: I often find myself cursing and swearing at myself, and this
is particularly the case when I am feeling tense in my
body

I've identified that my **DISCHARGER** is creating this controlled explosion:

HARM CREATED: *Attacks to switch on threat emotions and responses
(fight/flight)*

HARM AVERTED: *Pent-up emotions and undischarged responses may
cause disease*

Do I accept this? Do I want to address it? Or switch to a different strategy?

ACCEPT: Yes, I need to release this pent-up emotion stored in my
body and I accept that how my brain has been doing
that, through cursing and swearing at myself, is the way
I want to continue

ADDRESS: No, I don't want to curse and swear at myself anymore,
and yet I can feel my body is holding unresolved
emotional energy from the past. To address this, I first
want to understand what this emotion is (is it fear?
anger?) and go back to the initial memory where this
emotion had to be blocked or suppressed. This will
help me know how to feel and process this emotion
fully in its source context

SWITCH/DELAY: Yes, I need to release this pent-up emotion in my body
and I will take up boxing and just keep punching
people in the hope that this gets the emotion out of
my system

YOUR EXAMPLE. Self-criticism unit – DISCHARGER

SITUATION:

I've identified that my **DISCHARGER** is creating this controlled explosion:

HARM CREATED: ...

HARM AVERTED: ...

Do I accept this? Do I want to address it? Or switch to a different strategy?

ACCEPT:

ADDRESS:

SWITCH/DELAY:

Appendix 3.9   Self-criticism unit: SUBMITTER

SITUATION: When I go into a social situation, my self-critic attacks me and puts me down, which makes me feel small and inferior, and feel like I don't have anything useful to contribute

I've identified that my **SUBMITTER** is creating this controlled explosion:

HARM CREATED: *Self-critical attack elicits inferior feelings and submissive responses*

HARM AVERTED: *The likelihood of being a target of harm from other people*

Do I accept this? Do I want to address it? Or switch to a different strategy?

ACCEPT: Yes, I need to avoid every risk of being vulnerable to harm by others and I accept that how my self-critic has been keeping me in an inferior and submissive role is how I wish to continue this

ADDRESS: No, I don't want to self-criticise anymore, and yet I am aware of my fear of being a target and hurt again. To address this, I want to go back to process my early-life threats and traumas, and practise developing healthy assertiveness so that I can start showing up in the world as the person who I want to be

SWITCH/DELAY: Yes, I want to continue avoiding the risks of making myself a target, but rather than achieving self-submission through constant self-criticism, I will try and keep myself under the radar by self-sabotaging my career ambitions, goals, and contributions instead

YOUR EXAMPLE. Self-criticism unit – SUBMITTER

SITUATION:

I've identified that my **SUBMITTER** is creating this controlled explosion:

HARM CREATED: ...

HARM AVERTED: ...

Do I accept this? Do I want to address it? Or switch to a different strategy?

ACCEPT:

ADDRESS:

SWITCH/DELAY:

Appendix 3.10   Self-criticism unit: DISSOCIATOR

SITUATION: I have just quit my job because I couldn't cope with the stress, and I am attacking myself for being weak. I hate myself for being such a pathetic cry-baby and a loser
I've identified that my **DISSOCIATOR** is creating this controlled explosion:

HARM CREATED: *Attack or disown the 'needy' part of me*

HARM AVERTED: *The fear of being sad, vulnerable, weak, and small*

Do I accept this? Do I want to address it? Or switch to a different strategy?

ACCEPT: Yes, I want to disown these sad, weak, and vulnerable parts of me. They will only bring pain, and the way my brain's self-critic has learnt to attack them is the way to keep them out of my life

ADDRESS: No, I don't want to keep self-attacking and being hostile to these needy parts of me, and yet I can appreciate that being in touch with them is hard and will make me feel vulnerable. To address this, I want to start making space for more vulnerable feelings in my life. It might not have been safe to feel these emotions – and have these needs – as a child, but I am ready to start connecting with them now

SWITCH/DELAY: Yes, I do want to keep these sad and vulnerable parts of me at bay for now, because I am going through a lot of important changes in my life, and now is not the right time. I will keep using dissociation until I feel more settled in my life and am ready to open this up

YOUR EXAMPLE. Self-criticism unit – DISSOCIATOR

SITUATION:

I've identified that my **DISSOCIATOR** is creating this controlled explosion:

HARM CREATED: ...

HARM AVERTED: ...

Do I accept this? Do I want to address it? Or switch to a different strategy?

ACCEPT:

ADDRESS:

SWITCH/DELAY:

Appendix 3.11 Self-harm unit: MODIFIER

SITUATION: I am self-conscious about my appearance and have undergone some cosmetic procedures to change the shape and size of certain body parts to make me more attractive and desirable

I've identified that my **MODIFIER** is creating this controlled explosion:

> **HARM CREATED:** *Choosing to cause harm and pain by reconfiguring my body*

> **HARM AVERTED:** *Fear of being unattractive, undesirable, and socially isolated*

Do I accept this? Do I want to address it? Or switch to a different strategy?

ACCEPT: Yes, I do want to avoid these fears, and I accept that the strategy I have been using to achieve that by modifying my body is the one I wish to continue using

ADDRESS: No, I don't want to continue modifying my body from a place of fear, and yet I can see that there *are* underlying fears here linked to loneliness and isolation. To address this, I want to understand the fears more and where they have come from, so I can make wise choices (not purely from fear) about what I do with my body

SWITCH/DELAY: Yes, I do want to avoid these fears, but rather than doing so through reconfiguring my body on the outside, I will instead use dieting and exercising to bring about body changes from the inside

---

YOUR EXAMPLE. Self-harm unit – MODIFIER

SITUATION:

I've identified that my **MODIFIER** is creating this controlled explosion:

> **HARM CREATED:** ...

> **HARM AVERTED:** ...

Do I accept this? Do I want to address it? Or switch to a different strategy?

ACCEPT:

ADDRESS:

SWITCH/DELAY:

Appendix 3.12 Self-harm unit: REORIENTATOR

SITUATION: My body is feeling uncomfortable and bloated when I eat and I have been making myself vomit to feel less disgusting

I've identified that my **REORIENTATOR** is creating this controlled explosion:

HARM CREATED: *Forceful, self-induced vomiting*

HARM AVERTED: *Uncomfortable feeling of having 'bad' or excessive matter in my body*

Do I accept this? Do I want to address it? Or switch to a different strategy?

ACCEPT: Yes, I do want to avoid these uncomfortable feelings in my body, and making myself vomit is a self-controlled harm that I am prepared to go through to achieve this

ADDRESS: No, I don't want to keep purging my body like this, and yet I can see that I am struggling with the discomfort of feeling bad and disgusting when I eat. To address this, I want to get to the source of my disgust and shame feelings, and what memories they are linked to, so that these can be processed and linked back to past memories rather than to experiences in my day-to-day life now

SWITCH/DELAY: Yes, I do want to avoid these uncomfortable feelings in my body, but rather than forcing myself to vomit, I will instead try and distract and dissociate from my body through, e.g. fasting or drugs

---

YOUR EXAMPLE. Self-harm unit – REORIENTATOR

SITUATION:

I've identified that my **REORIENTATOR** is creating this controlled explosion:

HARM CREATED: ...

HARM AVERTED: ...

Do I accept this? Do I want to address it? Or switch to a different strategy?

ACCEPT:

ADDRESS:

SWITCH/DELAY:

Appendix 3.13   Self-harm unit: PAIN-RELIEVER

SITUATION: I have started scratching and cutting my skin, especially when I am feeling stressed and overwhelmed

I've identified that my **PAIN-RELIEVER** is creating this controlled explosion:

HARM CREATED: *Controlled physical pain. Body's natural pain relief systems initiated*

HARM AVERTED: *Emotional pain, suffering, torment that feels persistent and out of control*

Do I accept this? Do I want to address it? Or switch to a different strategy?

ACCEPT: Yes, it is important that I don't feel this emotional pain, and the strategy of causing physical harm to my body is something that I know comes with risks and is still the choice I am making

ADDRESS: No, I don't want to continue harming my body, and yet I am aware that my brain is fixed in a pattern of avoiding emotional pain. To address this, I know it will take time and courage, but developing compassionate understanding and care for my emotional suffering is a way I can break this pattern and move forward with my life

SWITCH/DELAY: Yes, I do want to avoid this emotional pain because I am not ready to face it yet. I will keep using this self-harming strategy as one of my resources while I build up a kitbag of other resources, and will decide later if I am ready to address this

YOUR EXAMPLE. Self-harm unit – PAIN-RELIEVER

SITUATION:

I've identified that my **PAIN-RELIEVER** is creating this controlled explosion:

HARM CREATED: ...

HARM AVERTED: ...

Do I accept this? Do I want to address it? Or switch to a different strategy?

ACCEPT:

ADDRESS:

SWITCH/DELAY:

Appendix 3.14 Self-harm unit: HABITUATOR

SITUATION: I was bullied at school, then got into bodybuilding. At the gym when I'm lifting heavy weights, I enjoy the aching muscles as this is a sign that I'm getting bigger and stronger. No pain no gain. You can't mess with me, and I can take anything you try to throw at me

I've identified that my **HABITUATOR** is creating this controlled explosion:

HARM CREATED: *Self-inflict pain as a preparatory measure to increase my general tolerance to/mastery over pain*

HARM AVERTED: *Being unprepared for and overwhelmed by pain from external events*

Do I accept this? Do I want to address it? Or switch to a different strategy?

ACCEPT: Yes, it is crucial that I have a high threshold and tolerance for pain, and that I put myself through this pain to get hardened and resilient

ADDRESS: No, I don't want to put my body through this pain anymore, and yet I'm aware that a big driver for me in my bodybuilding has been avoiding the fear of being weak and unprepared for bullies. To address this, I will get to the source of the fear (school) and develop some healthy protective anger around those experiences

SWITCH/DELAY: Yes, it is crucial that I avoid the risk of ever being hurt again by bullies who might hurt me, but rather than putting my body through these daily aches and pain, I will try to switch to another strategy such as being submissive (**SUBMITTER**) or self-blaming (**BLAMER**)

YOUR EXAMPLE. Self-harm unit – HABITUATOR

SITUATION:

I've identified that my **HABITUATOR** is creating this controlled explosion:

HARM CREATED: ...

HARM AVERTED: ...

Do I accept this? Do I want to address it? Or switch to a different strategy?

ACCEPT:

ADDRESS:

SWITCH/DELAY:

Appendix 3.15   Self-harm unit: CATALYST

SITUATION: I just wanted one doughnut on my walk back from work, but the shop only sold them in packs of five. I've eaten one and now I'm really stressed about whether or not I should have another

I've identified that my **CATALYST** is creating this controlled explosion:

> **HARM CREATED:** *I eat all the doughnuts and beat myself up to get it over and done with*
>
> **HARM AVERTED:** *Indefinite rumination, uncertainty, and anxious tension*

Do I accept this? Do I want to address it? Or switch to a different strategy?

ACCEPT: Yes, I want to stop feeling this uncertainty and anxious tension, so I accept this strategy as a way of arriving at a conclusion. I'll take the punishment now please and move on

ADDRESS: No, I don't want to catalyse this situation in a dramatic fashion for the sake of getting it over with, and yet I know my brain and body are struggling to stay with the tension. To address this, I will practise building my skills in distress tolerance and my courage to sit with uncertainty. There are some body posture, grounding, and breathing practices that I would like to try

SWITCH: Yes, I want to stop feeling this uncertainty and anxious tension, but rather than catalysing the situation, I am going to call on the **REORIENTATOR** to provide me with a diversion

---

YOUR EXAMPLE. Self-harm unit – CATALYST

SITUATION:

I've identified that my **CATALYST** is creating this controlled explosion:

HARM CREATED: ...

HARM AVERTED: ...

Do I accept this? Do I want to address it? Or switch to a different strategy?

ACCEPT:

ADDRESS:

SWITCH/DELAY:

Appendix 4

Controlled explosions imagery scripts

Appendices **4.1** to **4.7** are a series of imagery exercise scripts for compassionately engaging with your controlled explosions and the bomb squad members and 'selves' who are involved.

The first four scripts (**4.1** to **4.4**) are for *creating the conditions* for compassion, specifically creating a compassionate self and then preparing three scenes (*view from the balcony*; *room with chairs*; *calm place*) in which your compassionate self may be able to help:

4.1 Creating your *'ideal compassionate self'*
4.2 A *'view from the balcony'* scene
4.3 A *'room with chairs'* scene
4.4 A *'calm place'* scene.

The next three scripts (**4.5** to **4.7**) are for *using your compassionate self to meet a bomb squad member* who is creating a controlled explosion in your life, along with three of your different 'selves' (*day-to-day self; younger self; future self*) who may have useful insights to deepen your understanding of this controlled explosion and how to help:

4.5 Your *'day-to-day self'* who is being harmed by this controlled explosion
4.6 Your *'younger self'* who has been hurt in the past and is being protected by this controlled explosion
4.7 Your *'future self'* who has outgrown this controlled explosion.

These exercises will start with the same steps of preparing your body first (with grounded posture and breathing rhythm) and then connecting with the qualities of your compassionate self. When meeting a bomb squad member, as your compassionate self, you will first take the *'view from the balcony'* position to orientate yourself to the controlled explosion situation and to identify the different 'selves' that you will be inviting into your '*room with chairs*'.

If at any time during these exercises, something becomes difficult or feels too overwhelming, you can switch back to your '*calm place*' scene (Appendix **4.4**). The calm place is there whenever you need it, whether you'd like a temporary break from a meeting, with the intention of coming back, or whether you would like to close this meeting.

Appendix 4.1   Creating your 'ideal compassionate self'

Start by sitting in a comfortable, upright position, with feet flat on the floor ... and give your body a chance to settle into a posture that feels grounded, rooted, and stable ...

Now closing your eyes and dropping your awareness down into your body and your breath ... noticing the flow of your breathing in and out ... and just allowing your rhythm of breathing to settle in a smooth, even flow ... noticing those in-breaths coming deep down into the middle of your body ... and those long, smooth out-breaths ...

Easing your shoulders back slightly ... and creating a bit more expansiveness and volume in your chest ... and relaxing your facial muscles into a warm and friendly expression ...

Now create in your mind an image of your ideal compassionate self ... What do you imagine that would look like ... this version of you at your compassionate best? ... This is someone deeply committed to being a caring and helpful person ... and who brings these caring intentions into the world with a calm confidence, wisdom, and strength ...

Just noticing what that image looks like for a minute ... what you can see ... how they stand ... how they move ... the expression on their face ... and noticing what their voice tone sounds like when they speak ... Is there anything else you notice about them?

Now really focusing on some of the qualities of your ideal compassionate self ... qualities like wisdom, strength, and commitment to caring ... and as we go through each of these qualities, just notice how they come across in the image of your compassionate self ...

Caring-commitment ... How is this conveyed in the image of your compassionate self? Maybe through their facial expression, body language, or some other characteristic?

Wisdom ... How does this quality come across in the image? What is it about their mannerisms and expressions that show you they are wise ... that they have a deep understanding of people's struggles, and an intuitive knowledge of how to be helpful ...

Strength ... How does your compassionate self convey their inner strength and confidence in the image? Maybe there is something about their body language and movement which shows that they are anchored and grounded ... that they have the inner strength and courage to be a committed, caring, and compassionate person ...

Now that you've created your image, we're going to try stepping into the shoes of your compassionate self ... and imagine what that feels like becoming this person ... Just trying that for a minute ... being in the body and mind of your compassionate self ...

Noticing that inner calmness and strength in your body ... that wisdom and knowledge ... and what that feels like having a deep desire to be a caring and helpful person ...

Staying with that for a bit longer ... just connecting with that in your body and imagining what that feels like ... and imagining what that feels like looking out at the world through the eyes of your compassionate self ...

And when you're ready, you can bring this exercise to a close.

[Or instead of closing, if you are continuing with a practice of taking your compassionate self into one of the three scenes, you can continue straight from here into **4.2** to **4.4**]

Appendix 4.2   A *'view from the balcony'* scene

Staying anchored in the mind and body of your compassionate self, we're now going to imagine taking a 'view from the balcony' ... this is a view where you can see all the things that are going on ... like an ariel view ... You might think of this as similar to being up in the sky-box at a sports stadium, where you see all the players below you ... or maybe a wide-shot camera angle, where you can see things in the context of their environment ...

For this exercise, you are going to be up here on the balcony, as your compassionate self, and just spending a bit of time seeing yourself at home going through a typical day ...

Before we start, let's just check back in with your grounded body posture, your breathing rhythm, and the qualities of your compassionate self ... So here you are on the balcony ... the wise, strong, grounded version of you ... connected with that caring motivation of yours ... You want to be helpful and supportive ... You have a deep understanding of human struggles and what it's like to be a human with this tricky brain of ours ...

As you see yourself going through the motions of your day ... starting with waking up in the morning and getting out of bed ... you are holding a caring and supportive intention in your mind ... This person you see getting up is somebody that you care about ... somebody who you know struggles some days, just like everyone else ... It's not their fault ... You want to try and understand this person's struggles so that you can help ...

So from the balcony, just seeing yourself going through your morning routines ... maybe getting dressed, brushing your teeth ... making some breakfast or coffee ...

Just staying with that for a while longer, with your view from the balcony, looking through the lens of your wise and supportive compassionate self.

Appendix 4.3 A *'room with chairs'* scene

Staying anchored in the mind and body of your compassionate self, we're now going to imagine being in a room with some chairs … you can sit down in one chair, but the other chairs in front of you can remain empty for now … There will be various people coming to sit down with you here … sometimes just one person coming for an important conversation with you, sometimes it might be more of a gathering … For now, just make sure that your room is ready to welcome people as and when they arrive …

As your compassionate self, of course you care about people and their well-being … And just like a good host bringing guests into their home, it's important to you that people feel welcome, safe, and comfortable … that they feel looked after …

Hold in mind that sometimes people might be coming to talk to you about something difficult or painful … so what kind of environment can create safeness for them? …

As you imagine this room, what are some of the things you might see there to make this a more welcoming space? … Think about colours … objects … textures … lighting … What would this room look like if it was an *ideal* safe and comforting space? … What would the chairs look like? … How would they be arranged? … Just spend a bit more time looking around this room, getting a sense in your body of the safeness feeling that it's creating …

Appendix 4.4   A *'calm place'* scene

Staying anchored in the mind and body of your compassionate self, we're now going to imagine arriving in the scene of your ideal calm place … this could be any place you like … for example, a beach, a forest, a mountain, a garden, or a particular room in a house … It may be based on a real place you've been to before, or a place that's entirely made up … The main thing is that this place gives you a feeling of calmness and peacefulness …

When you have a sense of this, just take a look around this place, paying attention to what you can see… noticing any colours, shapes, objects … Notice what you can see close by to you, and what you can see further off in the distance … Now notice what you can hear … are there are any sounds in this place? … How does that feel for you being here in this calm place in amongst these sounds? … Notice whether there are any smells – maybe calming smells … Just notice these as you breathe calmly … and notice how these smells make you feel … Is there anything you can feel or touch in this place, such as the warmth of the sun on your skin, or the feel of grass or sand, or anything else there with you? …

Now just get a sense of your relationship to this calm place … Just as you are feeling content and happy to be in this place, this place is also happy that you are there … The place is glad that you have chosen it to be your calm place … It welcomes you there and is pleased to be able to support you to have these calm and peaceful feelings.

Appendix 4.5   Your 'day-to-day self' who is being harmed by this controlled explosion

[*Use the script in* **4.1** *to prepare your body and then connect with the qualities of your compassionate self*]

[*Use the script in* **4.2** *to arrive at your 'view from the balcony' scene*]

For this exercise, you are going to start up here on the balcony, as your compassionate self, and just spend a bit of time seeing yourself in a moment of your daily life when a controlled explosion is happening ... a moment of self-sabotaging, self-criticising or self-harming ... Imagine that you are seeing this happening now as you look down from your balcony ...

Notice where you are and what you are doing ... and see what happens as this controlled explosion is occurring in real time ... It might be a self-sabotaging behaviour, such as procrastinating or creating chaos ... It might be a moment where you are self-criticising or berating yourself ... It might be a situation where you are harming your body in some way, either on the inside – through food or substances – or on the outside ...

Once you have chosen the situation ... just watch this scene playing out from your balcony view ... and noticing some of the emotions, tensions, and conflicts that are involved ...

And as you see this happen, remembering to stay firmly anchored in your compassionate self ... as this wise and understanding version of you ... who is calm ... grounded ... and supportive ... As your compassionate self, you care about this person and their day-to-day struggles, and you want to help ...

We are now going to press *pause* on this scene ... and just think about which bomb squad member is present in this moment ... Which unit is it from? Is it Self-Sabotage? Self-Criticism? or Self-Harm? ... And which unit member specifically is there creating this controlled explosion for you? ... Is it the **CERTAINTY-SEEKER**? The **SUBMITTER**? The **PAIN-RELIEVER**? Or someone else? When you have identified the bomb squad member, you can invite them to come and join you for a meeting in your 'room with chairs'.

[*Use the script in* **4.3** *to arrive at your 'room with chairs' scene*]

You are sitting here now in your room with chairs, as your compassionate self ... You arrange the chairs in front of you so that there are two chairs facing you ... one is for the bomb squad member – who is creating the controlled explosion ... and the other is for your 'day-to-day' self – the version of you who is receiving this controlled explosion and being harmed by this in their daily life ...

You invite them to sit down ... You are welcoming, respectful, and thoughtful about their needs ... and as they settle down in their chairs, you are noticing if there's anything you can do – or offer – to help them feel more comfortable ... and if so, just do that now ...

As the compassionate self, you want to help, and you want to understand more about this conflict and why it's happening ... You want to understand about the deeper fears and concerns that might be driving this ...

But before you ask about this directly, just spend a minute longer resting with your deep compassionate intention towards them ... directing your compassion to this relationship and pattern they are caught in ... for the fears and emotions they are struggling with ... and directing towards them your desire to help them through this ...

When you're ready, you can ask the bomb squad member to tell you about why they are creating this harm or problem ... Maybe asking them directly: *"What is the reason for creating this?" "What are you afraid of?" "What would be your greatest fear if you couldn't create this controlled explosion?" "What are you protecting us from?"*

Once you have heard their response, you can then ask your 'day-to-day self' what that feels like for them being the recipient of this controlled explosion ...

Just stay with this conversation for another minute or two if you can, listening to both of them and hearing what they each have to say ... really tuning in to the emotions that are being felt, expressed, and communicated ... If at any point it strays into a battle or argument between them, just bring your attention back to posture, breathing, and using your calm presence and qualities to guide the conversation back to a collaborative process of discovery ... And remember you can use your 'calm place' image at any time you need ...

[As a prompt for some other directions you might want to take this conversation, there are a list of questions suggested on page 130 of Chapter 6 to ask your bomb squad member]

When they have finished speaking, you can calmly summarise and repeat back to them what you have heard ... You can also tell them what you have learnt about the function of the controlled explosion, and about the deeper fears and harms it is protecting ...

When speaking as the compassionate self, you are using your most warm and caring voice tone ... Your gestures and mannerisms are calm ... wise ... steady ... and supportive ...

If there is anything else that you think might be helpful to do or say to your day-to-day self, you can do that now ... something they may need to hear from you in this moment ... And just stay with that for a minute... directing your compassion to your day-to-day self ...

You can finish this exercise by returning to your 'view from the balcony', and seeing this scene below you, where your compassionate self is being supportive to your day-to-day self.

Appendix 4.6   Your *'younger self'* who has been hurt in the past and is being protected by this controlled explosion

[Use the script in **4.1** to prepare your body and then connect with the qualities of your compassionate self]

[Use the script in **4.2** to arrive at your 'view from the balcony' scene]

For this exercise, you are going to start up here on the balcony, as your compassionate self, and just spend a bit of time seeing your younger self … the younger version of you who was feeling vulnerable or hurt in some way … this is the hurt you have been avoiding with your controlled explosion …

And as you see this younger version of you, remembering to stay firmly anchored in your compassionate self … as this wise and understanding version of you … who is calm … grounded … and supportive … As your compassionate self, you care about this younger self and their struggles, and you want to help …

We are now going to press *pause* on this scene … and invite your younger self to come and join you for a meeting in your 'room with chairs'.

[Use the script in **4.3** to arrive at your 'room with chairs' scene]

You are sitting here now in your room with chairs, as your compassionate self … You arrange the chairs in front of you so that there are two chairs facing you … one is for the bomb squad member – who is creating the controlled explosion … and the other is for your 'younger' self – the version of you who has been hurt in the past and who the bomb squad member has been trying to protect with this controlled explosion …

You invite them to sit down … You are welcoming, respectful, and thoughtful about their needs … and as they settle down in their chairs, you are noticing if there's anything you can do – or offer – to help them feel more comfortable … and if so, just do that now …

As the compassionate self, you want to help, and you want to understand more about these harms experienced by your younger self, and why it was so important for these to be protected ... You want to understand how these underlying harms and fears may be linked to core needs of yours that were threatened or not met ...

But before you ask about this directly, just spend a minute longer resting with your deep compassionate intention towards them ... directing your compassion to this relationship pattern they are caught in ... for the fears and emotions they are struggling with ... and directing towards them your desire to help them through this ...

When you're ready, you can ask the younger self to tell you about their fears and their unmet needs ... Maybe asking them directly: *"What happened to you?" "What has hurt you?" "What are you scared of?" "What do you need?"*

Once you have heard their response, you can then bring in your bomb squad member and acknowledge the importance of the protective role they have played in relation to these younger experiences ...

Just stay with this conversation for another minute or two if you can, listening to both of them and hearing what they each have to say ... really tuning in to the emotions that are being felt, expressed, and communicated ... If at any point it strays into a battle or argument between them, just bring your attention back to posture, breathing, and using your calm presence and qualities to guide the conversation back to a collaborative process of discovery ... And remember you can use your 'calm place' image at any time you need ...

[As a prompt for some other directions you might want to take this conversation, there are a list of questions suggested on page 132 of Chapter 6 to ask your younger self]

When they have finished speaking, you can calmly summarise and repeat back to them what you have heard ... You can also tell them what you have learnt about the fears and harms, and about the basic needs that these are linked to ...

When speaking as the compassionate self, you are using your most warm and caring voice tone ... Your gestures and mannerisms are calm ... wise ... steady ... and supportive ...

If there is anything else that you think might be helpful to do or say to your younger self, you can do that now ... something they may need to feel – or hear – from you in this moment ... you might want to tell your younger self that it will be okay ... or maybe offer them some wisdom or guidance ... And just stay with that for a minute... directing your compassion to your younger self ...

You can finish this exercise by returning to your 'view from the balcony', and seeing this scene below you, where your compassionate self is taking care of your younger self.

Appendix 4.7   Your *'future self'* who has outgrown this controlled explosion

[Use the script in **4.1** to prepare your body and then connect with the qualities of your compassionate self]

[Use the script in **4.2** to arrive at your 'view from the balcony' scene]

For this exercise, you are going to start up here on the balcony, as your compassionate self, and just spend a bit of time seeing your future self ... the future version of you who has outgrown the fears of the younger self ... who has outgrown the need for using this controlled explosion in their life ...

See your future self going about their daily life ... Where are they? ... What does their environment look like? ... Any colours, smells, textures that you notice ... What do you notice about how this future version of you looks? ... What age they are ... What they are wearing ... What is their body language? ... their facial expression? ...

Observe them going about their daily motions and routines ... What do they do each day? ... How do they move and engage with what they are doing? ...

We are now going to press *pause* on this scene ... and invite your future self to come and join you for a meeting in your 'room with chairs' ...

[Use the script in **4.3** to arrive at your 'room with chairs' scene]

You are sitting here now in your room with chairs, as your compassionate self ... You arrange the chairs in front of you so that there are two chairs facing you ... one is for the bomb squad member – who has been creating this controlled explosion ... and the other is for your future self – the version of you who has outgrown this controlled explosion ...

You invite them to sit down ... You are welcoming, respectful, and thoughtful about their needs ... and as they settle down in their chairs, you are noticing if there's anything you can do – or offer – to help them feel more comfortable ... and if so, just do that now ...

As the compassionate self, you want to learn, and you want to understand more about the process that your future self has gone through to outgrow the fear and the controlled explosion ... You want to understand what old structures and patterns they have let go of, and what new structures they have built in their place ... You want to ask them what their new life looks like ... and what's different and good about it ...

But before you ask about this directly, just spend a minute longer resting with your deep compassionate intention towards them ... directing your compassion to their relationship and what they have worked through together ... the journey they've been on ... recognising that change does not come easily, and often involves sacrifices ... appreciating their courage and strength ...

When you're ready, you can ask the future self to tell you about their life ... Maybe asking them directly: *"What new structures and routines have you built?" "What did you have to let go of to get to where you are now?" "What advice would you give?"*

Once you have heard their response, you can then bring in your bomb squad member and ask them if listening to the future self has helped them to feel safe ... and if there is anything else they need to hear from them to feel more safe ... safe enough to let go of control ...

Just stay with this conversation for another minute or two if you can, listening to both of them and hearing what they each have to say ... really tuning in to the emotions that are being felt, expressed, and communicated ... If at any point it strays into a battle or argument between them, just bring your attention back to posture, breathing, and using your calm presence and qualities to guide the conversation back to a collaborative process of discovery ... And remember you can use your 'calm place' image at any time you need ...

[As a prompt for some other directions you might want to take this conversation, there are a list of questions suggested on page 142 of Chapter 6 to ask your future self]

When they have finished speaking, you can calmly summarise and repeat back to them what you have heard ... You can tell them what you have learnt about their processes of growth and transformation ... of outgrowing their old fears and letting go of things that were no longer working for them ... and expanding their brain and world to accommodate the new things that they've always really wanted and needed in their life ...

When speaking as the compassionate self, you are using your most warm and caring voice tone ... Your gestures and mannerisms are calm ... wise ... steady ... and supportive ...

If there is anything else that you might like to do – or say – to your future self, you can do that now … something they may like to hear from you in this moment … you might want to tell them that you admire their strength and courage … That you are proud of how they have shown up in their life and taken these important steps forward … And just stay with that for a minute … directing your compassion to your future self …

You can finish this exercise by returning to your 'view from the balcony', and seeing this scene below you, where your compassionate self is happy and proud of your future self.

Appendix 5

Resources for self-understanding and self-help

Self-understanding/Self-help books

- *Emotional Difficulties* – Chris Irons [70]
- *Beating Overeating* – Ken Goss [42]
- *Recovering from Trauma* – Deborah Lee [71]
- *Managing your Anger* – Russell Kolts [72]
- *Building your Self-confidence* – Mary Welford [73]
- *Overcoming Anxiety* – Dennis Tirch [74]
- *Relating to Voices* – Charlie Heriot-Maitland and Eleanor Longden [14]

Other recommended books

- *The Art of Losing Control* – Jules Evans [65]
- *When You're Falling, Dive* – Mark Matousek [43]
- *Good Reasons for Bad Feelings* – Randolph Nesse [1]
- *The Compassionate Mind* – Paul Gilbert [41]
- *Why Love Matters* – Sue Gerhardt [75]
- *Trauma and Recovery* – Judith Herman [76]
- *Memories, Dreams, Reflections* – Carl Jung [77]

Compassion Focused Therapy websites

- *Balanced Minds* – Therapy practice, training, resources (www.balanced minds.com)
- *Compassionate Mind Foundation* – Training, info. (www.compassionatemind. co.uk)

Podcast

- *This Jungian Life* (www.thisjungianlife.com)

Ted Talks

- *The Voices in My Head* – Eleanor Longden [78]
- *Do We See Reality as It Is?* – Donald Hoffman [6]

Author's personal website

- www.charlieheriotmaitland.com

References

1. Nesse, R.M. (2019). *Good reasons for bad feelings: Insights from the frontier of evolutionary psychiatry.* Penguin.
2. Shepard, R.N. (1990). *Mind sights: Original visual illusions, ambiguities, and other anomalies, with a commentary on the play of mind in perception and art.* WH Freeman/Times Books/Henry Holt & Co.
3. Adelson, E.H. (1995). *Checkershadow illusion.* https://persci.mit.edu/gallery/checkershadow
4. Skye, V. (2017). *Skye Blue Cafe Wall Illusion.* 2017 (cited 2025); www.youtube.com/watch?v=d8Se0WRFV-8&t=2s
5. Lotto, B. (2018). *Deviate: The creative power of transforming your perception.* Weidenfeld & Nicolson.
6. Hoffman, D. (2015) *Do we see reality as it is?* [Online Video]. TED 2015: www.ted.com/talks/donald_hoffman_do_we_see_reality_as_it_is?language=en
7. Clark, A. (2013). Whatever next? Predictive brains, situated agents, and the future of cognitive science. *Behavioral & Brain Sciences, 36*(3), 181–204.
8. Friston, K. and Kiebel, S. (2009). Predictive coding under the free-energy principle. *Philosophical Transactions of the Royal Society B: Biological Sciences, 364*(1521): 1211–1221.
9. Wilkinson, S., Dodgson, G., & Meares, K. (2017). Predictive processing and the varieties of psychological trauma. *Frontiers in Psychology, 8,* 1840.
10. Seth, A. (2021). *Being you: A new science of consciousness.* Penguin.
11. Heriot-Maitland, C., & Bell, T. (2025). Compassion-focused chairwork for voice-hearing relationships, body triggers and motivational states. *Psychology and Psychotherapy: Theory, Research, and Practice,* https://doi.org/10.1111/papt.12600
12. van Os, J., Linscott, R.J., Myin-Germeys, I., Delespaul, P., & Krabbendam, L. (2009). A systematic review and meta-analysis of the psychosis continuum: Evidence for a psychosis proneness-persistence-impairment model of psychotic disorder. *Psychological Medicine, 39*(2), 179–195.
13. Flor, H. (2002). Phantom-limb pain: Characteristics, causes, and treatment. *Lancet Neurology, 1*(3): 182–189.
14. Heriot-Maitland, C., & Longden, E. (2022). *Relating to voices using compassion focused therapy: A self-help companion.* Routledge.
15. Callan, M.J., Kay, A.C., & Dawtrey, R.J. (2014). Making sense of misfortune: deservingness, self-esteem, and patterns of self-defeat. *Journal of Personality and Social Psychology, 107*(1), 142–162.

16. Klayman, J. (1995). Varieties of confirmation bias. *Psychology of Learning and Motivation, 32*, 385–418.

17. Lerner, M.J. (1980). *The belief in a just world: A fundamental delusion.* Springer.

18. Sherman, D.K., & Cohen, G.L. (2006). The psychology of self-defense: Self-affirmation theory. *Advances in Experimental Social Psychology, 38*, 183–242.

19. Jussim, L. (1986). Self-fulfilling prophecies: A theoretical and integrative review. *Psychological Review, 93*(4), 429.

20. De Boer, H., Timmermans, A.C., & Van Der Werf, M.P. (2018). The effects of teacher expectation interventions on teachers' expectations and student achievement: Narrative review and meta-analysis. *Educational Research and Evaluation, 24*(3–5), 180–200.

21. Chen, M., & Bargh, J.A. (1997). Nonconscious behavioral confirmation processes: The self-fulfilling consequences of automatic stereotype activation. *Journal of Experimental Social Psychology, 33*(5), 541–560.

22. Dweck, C. (2015). Carol Dweck revisits the growth mindset. *Education Week, 35*(5), 20–24.

23. Curtis, R.C., & Miller, K. (1986). Believing another likes or dislikes you: Behaviors making the beliefs come true. *Journal of Personality and Social Psychology, 51*(2), 284.

24. Petropoulos Petalas, D., van Schie, H., & Hendriks Vettehen, P. (2017). Forecasted economic change and the self-fulfilling prophecy in economic decision-making. *PLoS One, 12*(3), e0174353.

25. Miller, M., White, B., & Scrivner, C. (2024). Surfing uncertainty with screams: predictive processing, error dynamics and horror films. *Philosophical Transactions of the Royal Society B: Biological Sciences, 379*(1895), 20220425.

26. Lubart, T.I., & Getz, I. (1997). Emotion, metaphor, and the creative process. *Creativity Research Journal, 10*(4), 285–301.

27. Grylls, B. (2013). *A survival guide for life.* Random House.

28. Lucre, K. (2025). *Compassion focused group psychotherapy: An exploratory programme for people who could have a diagnosis of 'personality'.* Pavilion Publishing and Media Ltd.

29. Gilbert, P., & Simos, G. (2022). Compassion focused therapy, in *Compassion Focused Therapy* (pp. 24–89). Routledge.

30. Linscott, R.J., & van Os, J. (2013). An updated and conservative systematic review and meta-analysis of epidemiological evidence on psychotic experiences in children and adults: On the pathway from proneness to persistence to dimensional expression across mental disorders. *Psychological Medicine, 43*(6), 1133–1149.

31. Heriot-Maitland, C., Knight, M., & Peters, E. (2012). A qualitative comparison of psychotic-like phenomena in clinical and non-clinical populations. *British Journal of Clinical Psychology, 51*(1), 37–53.

32. Jackson, M., & Fulford, K. (2002). Psychosis good and bad: Values-based practice and the distinction between pathological and nonpathological forms of psychotic experience. *Philosophy, Psychiatry, & Psychology, 9*(4), 387–394.

33. Gilbert, P. (2005). Social mentalities: A biopsychosocial and evolutionary approach to social relationships, in M.W. Baldwin (Ed.), *Interpersonal Cognition.* Guilford Press.

34. Gilbert, P., Clarke, M., Hempel, S., Miles, J.N.V., & Irons, C. (2004). Criticizing and reassuring oneself: An exploration of forms, styles and reasons in female students. *British Journal of Clinical Psychology, 43*(Pt 1), 31–50.

35. Maté, G. (2011). *When the body says no: The cost of hidden stress.* Vintage Canada.

36. Sieff, D.F. (2017). Trauma-worlds and the wisdom of Marion Woodman. *Psychological Perspectives*, *60*(2), 170–185.
37. Taylor, P.J., Gooding, P., Wood, A.M., & Tarrier, N. (2011). The role of defeat and entrapment in depression, anxiety, and suicide. *Psychological Bulletin*, *137*(3), 391–420.
38. Kalsched, D. (2018). *Unlocking the secrets of the wounded psyche: The miraculous survival system that is also a prison*, D. Sieff (Ed.). https://danielasieff.com/wp-content/uploads/2021/08/Sieff-Kalsched-2008-Unlocking-the-Secrets-of-the-Wounded-Psyche-compressed.pdf
39. Wohlrab, S., Stahl, J., & Kappeler, P.M. (2007). Modifying the body: Motivations for getting tattooed and pierced. *Body Image*, *4*(1), 87–95.
40. de Berker, A.O., Rutledge, R.B., Mathys, C., Marshall, L., Cross, G.F., Dolan, R.J., & Bestmann, S. (2016). Computations of uncertainty mediate acute stress responses in humans. *Nature Communications*, *7*(1), 10996.
41. Gilbert, P. (2009). *The compassionate mind: A new approach to facing the challenges of life*. Constable & Robinson.
42. Goss, K. (2011). *The compassionate mind approach to beating overeating*. Constable & Robinson.
43. Matousek, M. (2011). *When you're falling, dive: Lessons in the art of living*. Bloomsbury Publishing USA.
44. Heriot-Maitland, C. (2011). Multi-level models of information processing, and their application to psychosis. *Journal of Experimental Psychopathology*, *3*(4), 552–571.
45. Clarke, I. (2008). Pioneering a cross-diagnostic approach founded in cognitive science, in *Cognitive behaviour therapy for acute inpatient mental health units* (pp. 83–94). Routledge.
46. Freeman, D. (2007). Suspicious minds: The psychology of persecutory delusions. *Clinical Psychology Review*, *27*(4), 425–457.
47. Seth, A.K. (2013). Interoceptive inference, emotion, and the embodied self. *Trends in Cognitive Science*, *17*(11), 565–573.
48. Gilbert, P. (2009). Introducing compassion-focused therapy. *Advances in Psychiatric Treatment*, *15*(3), 199–208.
49. Gilbert, P. (2014). The origins and nature of compassion focused therapy. *British Journal of Clinical Psychology*, *53*(1), 6–41.
50. Gilbert, P., & Simos, G. (2022). *Compassion focused therapy: Clinical practice and applications*. Routledge.
51. Gilbert, P., & Procter, S. (2006). Compassionate mind training for people with high shame and self-criticism: Overview and pilot study of a group therapy approach. *Clinical Psychology & Psychotherapy: An International Journal of Theory & Practice*, *13*(6), 353–379.
52. Irons, C., & Beaumont, E. (2017). *The compassionate mind workbook: A step-by-step guide to developing your compassionate self*. Constable & Robinson.
53. Irons, C., & Heriot-Maitland, C. (2021). Compassionate mind training: An 8-week group for the general public. *Psychological Psychotherapy*, *94*(3), 443–463.
54. Geller, S.M., & Porges, S.W. (2014). Therapeutic presence: Neurophysiological mechanisms mediating feeling safe in therapeutic relationships. *Journal of Psychotherapy Integration*, *24*(3), 178–192.
55. Porges, S.W. (2007). The polyvagal perspective. *Biological Psychology*, *74*(2), 116–143.
56. Dana, D. (2018). *The Polyvagal theory in therapy: Engaging the rhythm of regulation* (Norton series on interpersonal neurobiology). WW Norton.

57. Petrocchi, N., & Cheli, S. (2019). The social brain and heart rate variability: Implications for psychotherapy. *Psychological Psychotherapy, 92*(2), 208–223.
58. Matos, M., Duarte, C., de Matos Duarte, J., Pinto-Gouveia, J., Petrocchi, N., Basran, J., & Gilbert, P. (2017). Psychological and physiological effects of compassionate mind training: A pilot randomised controlled study. *Mindfulness, 8*(6), 1699–1712.
59. Kirby, J.N., Doty, J., Petrocchi, N., & Gilbert, P. (2017). The current and future role of heart rate variability for assessing and training compassion. *Frontiers in Public Health, 5*, 40.
60. Di Bello, M., Ottaviani, C., & Petrocchi, N. (2021). Compassion is not a benzo: Distinctive associations of heart rate variability with its empathic and action components. *Frontiers in Neuroscience, 15*, 223.
61. Di Bello, M., Petrocchi, N., & Ottaviani, C. (2020). The compassionate vagus: A meta-analysis on the connection between compassion and heart rate variability. *Neuroscience & Biobehavioral Reviews, 116*, 21–30.
62. Walker, M. (2017). *Why we sleep: Unlocking the power of sleep and dreams.* Simon & Schuster.
63. Heriot-Maitland, C. (2008). Mysticism and madness: Different aspects of the same human experience? *Mental Health, Religion & Culture, 11*(3), 301–308.
64. Batson, C.D., & Ventis, W.L. (1982). *The religious experience: A social-psychological perspective.* Oxford University Press.
65. Evans, J. (2017). *The art of losing control: A philosopher's search for ecstatic experience.* Canongate Books.
66. Heriot-Maitland, C., & Taylor, J. (2023). *Compassionate parenting* [online course]. https://compassioncourses.com/compassionate-parenting.
67. ITV (2022). *Trigger Point* [television series]
68. Ofcom (2023). *Top trends from our latest Media Nations research.*
69. Heriot-Maitland, C., Vitoratu, S., Peters, E., Hermans, K., Wykes, T., & Brett, C. (2023). Detecting anomalous experiences in the community: The Transpersonal Experiences Questionnaire (TEQ). *Psychological Psychotherapy, 96*(2), 383–398.
70. Irons, C. (2019). *The compassionate mind approach to difficult emotions: Using compassion focused therapy.* Constable & Robinson.
71. Lee, D., & James, S. (2012). *The compassionate mind approach to recovering from trauma: Using compassion focused therapy.* Hachette UK.
72. Kolts, R. (2012). *The compassionate mind approach to managing your anger: Using compassion-focused therapy.* Hachette UK.
73. Welford, M. (2012). *The compassionate mind approach to building self-confidence*: Series editor, Paul Gilbert. Constable & Robinson.
74. Tirch, D. (2012). *The compassionate mind approach to overcoming anxiety: Using compassion-focused therapy.* Hachette UK.
75. Gerhardt, S. (2014). *Why love matters: How affection shapes a baby's brain.* Routledge.
76. Herman, J.L. (2015). *Trauma and recovery: The aftermath of violence – from domestic abuse to political terror.* Hachette UK.
77. Jung, C.G. (1989). *Memories, dreams, reflections,* Vol. 268. Vintage.
78. Longden, E. (2013). *The voices in my head* [online video]. www.ted.com/talks/eleanor_longden_the_voices_in_my_head?language=en

Index

For Product Safety Concerns and Information please contact our EU
representative GPSR@taylorandfrancis.com
Taylor & Francis Verlag GmbH, Kaufingerstraße 24, 80331 München, Germany